W9-BLE-131

"Complete, accurate, and contemporary ... the *Interstitial Cystitis Survival Guide* will serve as an excellent reference for not only the patient, but also those clinicians who are interested in treating this disease. Every aspect of this difficult clinical problem is discussed in depth with clear and concise organization. This is an excellent reference book answering many of the questions that arise both from physicians and patients. Certainly, this is a much-needed book that will inform many patients and assist the treating physician with modern thoughts and theories regarding etiology and treatment."

—S. Grant Mulholland, M.D., Professor and Chairman, Department of Urology, Thomas Jefferson Medical College

THE

INTERSTITIAL CYSTITIS

SURVIVAL GUIDE

Your Guide to the Latest Treatment
Options and Coping Strategies

Robert M. Moldwin, M.D., F.A.C.S.

New Harbinger Publications, Inc.

Publisher's Note

Care has been taken to confirm the accuracy of the information presented and to describe generally accepted practices. However, the authors, editors, and publisher are not responsible for errors or omissions or for any consequences from application of the information in this book and make no warranty, express or implied, with respect to the contents of the publication.

The authors, editors, and publisher have exerted every effort to ensure that any drug selection and dosage set forth in this text are in accordance with current recommendations and practice at the time of publication. However, in view of ongoing research, changes in government regulations, and the constant flow of information relating to drug therapy and drug reactions, the reader is urged to check the package insert for each drug for any change in indications and dosage and for added warnings and precautions. This is particularly important when the recommended agent is a new or infrequently employed drug.

Some drugs and medical devices presented in this publication may have Food and Drug Administration (FDA) clearance for limited use in restricted research settings. It is the responsibility of the health care provider to ascertain the FDA status of each drug or device planned for use in their clinical practice.

Distributed in the U.S.A. by Publishers Group West; in Canada by Raincoast Books; in Great Britain by Airlift Book Company, Ltd.; in South Africa by Real Books, Ltd.; in Australia by Boobook; and in New Zealand by Tandem Press.

Copyright © 2000 by Robert M. Moldwin
        New Harbinger Publications, Inc.
        5674 Shattuck Avenue
        Oakland, CA 94609

Cover design © 2000 by Lightbourne Images
Edited by Kayla Sussell
Illustrations by Robert Moldwin, M.D.
Text design by Tracy Marie Powell

ISBN 1-57224-210-8 Paperback

All Rights Reserved

Printed in the United States of America

New Harbinger Publications' Web site address: www.newharbinger.com

02   01   00

10   9   8   7   6   5   4   3   2   1

First printing

To my wife, Rebecca, and to my children Elissa, Tracy, and Daniel, for all their wholehearted encouragement, support, and understanding while this book was being written. Rebecca—you always wanted me to write this book—well, here it is!

To my patients: There's no better motivation in medicine than to see a patient's life change for the better. My patients are my driving force in this field and in my writing.

—Robert M. Moldwin

Contents

Acknowledgments

I would like to acknowledge the many individuals who have been instrumental in the development of my career and in the writing of *The Interstitial Cystitis Survival Guide*.

To my dear friends and mentors, Dr. S. Grant Mulholland and Dr. Dolores Shupp-Byrne, of Thomas Jefferson Medical College. Thank you for introducing me to the realm of interstitial cystitis (IC) and for continuing to support my work.

To Dr. C. Lowell Parsons, Dr. Grannum Sant, and Dr. Phillip Hanno. Thank you for warmly welcoming me into the IC research community. Your pioneering research in IC continues to be a model for me and for other investigators.

Thanks to the caring and devoted staff of the Interstitial Cystitis Association (ICA). I greatly appreciate the time and effort that Dr. Vicky Ratner, President of the ICA, put into writing her comprehensive chapter, Support for the interstitial cystitis Patient.

Many thanks to Nancy Taylor, current Executive Director of the ICA and Debra Slade, past Executive Director of the ICA, for allowing me to become an integral part of their organization. I owe a special debt of gratitude to Lucretia Perilli, the ICA's medical communications specialist and the associate editor of the *ICA Update*. Her insight and incredible fund of knowledge has helped immeasurably in writing this book.

I wish to thank my institution, The North Shore–Long Island Jewish Health System, and specifically the Chairman of Urology, Dr. Arthur D. Smith. He has been an inspiration to me since medical school days and he continues to be my constant advisor and advocate. Many thanks to our terrific nurses, medical assistants, technicians, and secretaries who staff our Interstitial Cystitis Treatment Center. In particular, I wish to recognize Nancy Brettschneider, C.U.R.N., and Francine Mendelowitz, C.S.W. These two colleagues truly give their all to the physical and emotional well-being of our IC patients.

It is to New Harbinger Press' great credit to publish the first book exclusively written for the interstitial cystitis patient. Much of this credit specifically goes to Jueli Gastwirth and Kristin Beck, both of whom have always been enthusiastic supporters. I'd also like to send a heartfelt thanks to my editor, Kayla Sussell, for her tireless efforts and unique ability at keeping me on schedule.

Introduction

Doris M., a forty-one-year-old kindergarten teacher, wife, and mother of two, would never forget the spring morning in 1985 that changed her life forever. As she finished her daily mug of hot coffee, Doris experienced a twinge of discomfort in her lower abdomen. She tried to put the strange, annoying sensation out of her mind but it just wouldn't leave. Instead, it seemed to intensify a bit and she felt the urge to urinate. When she went to the bathroom, however, she produced only a small amount of urine, but some of the discomfort disappeared. As she dressed for work, she thought, "Well I guess I'm okay," but the miserable sensation returned and seemed even worse than before. "I must have a bladder infection," she thought. "I'd better call my doctor."

Doris was able to make an appointment with her internist, Dr. Davis, for later that day. Deciding to try to follow her normal routine, she made her way to work. The children in the kindergarten didn't see much of Doris that day because she disappeared into the bathroom every half hour. "I'm beginning to feel like I live in here," she thought.

Dr. Davis agreed that Doris probably had a bladder infection, which he referred to as "bacterial cystitis." He sent a urinalysis and urine culture off to the lab and prescribed a course of antibiotic therapy.

Doris suffered the longest, most sleepless night of her life. Bleary-eyed, she went to work the next morning believing that, with antibiotics in her system, her condition would improve. Two days later, though, she was still urinating every half hour, day and night.

Her husband, Ted, was becoming concerned and was not getting much sleep either.

The lab reports showed no signs of infection, but Doris was still feeling just awful. Dr. Davis prescribed a different antibiotic but to no avail—her symptoms persisted and dread began to overwhelm her. Back in the doctor's office she asked, "Is it possible that I have cancer?" "I doubt that," Dr. Davis replied, "but let's run some additional tests to exclude other medical problems that might account for your symptoms." No abnormalities were found. Perplexed, Dr. Davis referred Doris to a urologist for a consultation.

Doris' subsequent odyssey through the medical system took her through evaluations by three urologists and two gynecologists. The last doctor suggested, "You need to relax. Maybe you should see a psychologist since your symptoms seem to be stress-related." Indeed, Doris was stressed. Both going to and coming home from work each day, she had to stop twice on the road to urinate. Fatigue from loss of sleep was taking a staggering toll on her family life and her career. Her constant pelvic pain waxed and waned and frequently prevented her from participating in family gatherings. Sexual intercourse was not only uncomfortable—it worsened her symptoms for the rest of the week. She felt as though her life was falling apart bit by bit. Ted was very supportive, but he couldn't prevent Doris from falling into clinical depression.

This terribly distressing scenario is quite typical of many patients who are later found to have *interstitial cystitis (IC)*, a disease characterized by the need to urinate frequently and urgently. In most instances, it is accompanied by pelvic discomfort (or outright pain). Unfortunately, the correct diagnosis is often overlooked. This is because most patients show no specific findings upon physical examination or laboratory testing.

Even office cystoscopy (examining the bladder wall with a long, skinny telescope-like instrument called a cystoscope) usually fails to demonstrate any abnormalities. The average patient with interstitial cystitis sees three to five physicians and suffers for approximately three to seven years before a correct diagnosis is made. By then, many patients have become disgusted with the entire traditional medical system. They either pursue alternative, nonallopathic forms of care or they just suffer silently. As in Doris' case, the impact of the disease on sexual relations, family life, work, and the limitations of travel often result in clinical depression. Suicide is not unknown in this patient group.

As horrific as this story might seem, situations such as Doris' still occur, albeit less frequently these days. Over the past ten to fifteen years, medical ignorance regarding IC has slowly waned. We now realize that it is not rare at all. In fact, the most recent epidemiological studies indicate that there are approximately 700,000 people in the United States afflicted with IC right now (Curhan, Speizer, Hunter, Curhan, et al. 1999). More people have IC than hemophilia A, (Rodgers and Greenberg 1999), multiple sclerosis (Adams, Maurice, and Ropper 1997a), lupus (Gladman and Hochberg 1999) or Duchenne muscular dystrophy (Adams, Maurice, and Ropper 1997b).

Today, IC research, often sponsored by federal funding, has provided some much-needed information about aspects of the disease ranging from possible viral causes to associated immunological abnormalities. These data have given patients and their caregivers a much better understanding of the mechanisms of the disease and have opened the door to potentially new treatment strategies. Private industry has come to the aid of the IC patient, spending millions of dollars on research, pharmaceutical development, and physician education. The media has also been of great assistance to the IC patient as evidenced by numerous newspaper and magazine articles, and television stories.

The vast majority of these advances in understanding the illness have been made possible through the extraordinary efforts of the Interstitial Cystitis Association (ICA). This patient advocacy group has led a tireless campaign on behalf of the IC patient since 1984. Their work has included lobbying efforts in Washington, D.C., patient support groups, doctor referral networks, and the dissemination of patient literature. They have even generated funding of their own to sponsor IC-directed research. The ICA is discussed in greater detail in chapter 11.

The primary objective of this book is to build a framework for delivering proper care to the IC patient. The text emphasizes methods to diagnose IC and is heavily weighted toward treatment strategies. Please keep in mind while reading that *the diagnosis and management of IC is an ever-evolving process* and that *strategies to care for the IC patient may vary considerably from doctor to doctor*. Although our general treatment protocols will be outlined, this does not imply that other forms of care are wrong or are not as successful. Careful attention has been paid to provide as evenhanded an approach as possible to the many forms of care that are available. Lastly, remember that *this book is meant to serve as a helpful guide and not as a substitute for a qualified, empathetic caregiver*.

Chapter 1

Interstitial Cystitis 101: The Basics

Cystitis is a very nonspecific term meaning inflammation of the bladder. When most people (including doctors) think about cystitis, infection of the bladder comes to mind. That's because by far the most common form of cystitis is caused by bacteria and is aptly called *bacterial cystitis*. Interstitial cystitis (IC), on the other hand, does not appear to be related to infection.

The term "interstitial cystitis" was first used by A. J. C. Skene (1887) who described a disease of the urinary bladder marked by inflammation and ulceration (interstitial cystitis means inflammation (*cystitis*) within (*interstitial*) the bladder wall). In 1915, Dr. Guy Hunner described specific gross and microscopic details about these ulcers and the ulcers ultimately became known by his name (Hunner's ulcers). Today the criteria by which we make a diagnosis of interstitial cystitis have significantly broadened. *We now make the diagnosis of IC based upon oversensitivity of the bladder, whether or not inflammation of the bladder wall is present.*

As suggested in the Introduction, interstitial cystitis is a disease recognized by its symptoms. There are no specific blood or urine tests that firmly tell a clinician whether IC is present or not. Rather, the diagnosis is made on a "clinical" basis. This means that the physician reviews your medical history, your physical exam, and other tests (see chapter 2, Diagnosing Interstitial Cystitis) to make a final diagnosis. Much of the testing of an IC patient involves making sure that no other disease is present that might cause identical symptoms. In fact, the diagnosis of IC has often been termed "a diagnosis of exclusion."

The average IC patient's symptoms begin between thirty and fifty years of age; however, IC has been reported both in early childhood and in later adult life. Usually, the symptoms appear suddenly and initially are often confused with a bladder infection. Many patients actually remember the exact moment or date of symptom onset. Nonresponse to antibiotic treatment at this point should alert the clinician to the possibility of IC as a diagnosis. The symptoms of IC usually plateau and then tend to wax and wane. Spontaneous remissions (*we all love when this happens*) may occur but, unfortunately, symptoms often return weeks to months later. Urinary incontinence is rarely associated with IC. When it does occur, it is often associated with abnormal bladder contractions, a condition called "the overactive bladder" or "detrusor (bladder) instability."

About 90 percent of interstitial cystitis patients are women. This statistic might change in the future. We are currently discovering that many men previously diagnosed with certain forms of prostatitis actually have IC. This is a very exciting possibility since these patients generally have had a poor response to most therapies. The diagnosis of IC may open the door to new therapeutic options for these patients (see chapter 7, The Male with Interstitial Cystitis).

The question of a genetic component to IC remains unanswered. In most instances, no family history of bladder complaints exists. However, clinicians do occasionally see family members with IC. It has also been seen in identical twins. The mere fact that IC is more prevalent in females also suggests some genetic link.

Different Types of Interstitial Cystitis

Interstitial cystitis has been divided into two different categories, "classical" (or "ulcerative") disease and "nonclassical" (or "nonulcerative) disease". The classical, ulcerated form is the type that was originally described and associated with red patches of inflammation, called Hunner's ulcers. Classical IC is found in less than 10 percent of patients. Patients having these ulcers tend to have more severe symptoms. They also tend to have scarring of the bladder wall and, therefore, their bladder capacity slowly diminishes over time. In our experience, they are usually older than those with the nonulcerative disease. As you can imagine, the presence of typical symptoms and a bladder ulcer makes the diagnosis of IC quite simple, but, as mentioned, patients with nonulcerative disease are seen far more commonly. In the nonulcerated form of the illness, no specific lesions are noted upon routine bladder inspection.

There is a wide range in the severity of disease. For example, many patients awaken one or two times a night to urinate, whereas other patients need a bedside commode to deal with needing to void every fifteen minutes. Some patients describe the pain as an uncomfortable pressure above their pubic bone that is somewhat relieved by urinating. Others are completely incapacitated by pain to the point where simply walking to the bathroom is a monumental effort.

Recognizing the Symptoms of Interstitial Cystitis

The three most common symptoms of IC are:

* Frequency of urination

* Urgency of urination

* Pelvic pain; often worsening with the bladder filling and lessening with the bladder emptying

In 1993, Koziol, Clark, Gittes, and Tan studied 374 patients with IC. They noted that urinary frequency was the most commonly reported complaint and was present in about 92 percent of patients. Urinary urgency, the sudden need to void, was reported in about 89 percent of patients. Pelvic pain, pressure, and/or "bladder spasms" was seen in over 60 percent of patients. Unfortunately, the list of problems doesn't stop here.

Other commonly reported symptoms include the following:

* Pelvic pain worsening one week prior to the menstrual period

* Constipation or irritable bowel syndrome

* Slow urinary stream

* Pain with sexual intercourse or increased pelvic pain occurring twelve to twenty-four hours after sexual intercourse

* Depression

* Pain at the tip of the penis, the groin, or in the testicles in male patients

* Worsening of symptoms with certain foods or beverages

* Urethral burning (the *urethra* is the tube that carries urine out of the body)

In conclusion, interstitial cystitis can be generally defined as an oversensitivity of the bladder. There's a wide range of symptom severity. Some patients with the mildest forms of IC probably don't even visit their doctors. They live with their symptoms and make changes in their lifestyles to deal with their discomfort. On the other hand, there exists a huge number of afflicted individuals whose whole lives revolve around their bladders. Interstitial cystitis has reduced their quality of life considerably. Although we don't have a cure for IC, we do have many therapies that can significantly help many of these people. But, as you'll see in the next chapter, before any therapy can begin, it's important to have the right diagnosis.

Chapter 2

Diagnosing Interstitial Cystitis

You may ask at this point, "Do I have interstitial cystitis (IC) if I have some pelvic discomfort and go to the bathroom a lot." The answer is an emphatic "possibly, but not necessarily!" These symptoms are certainly suggestive of IC, but your physician would need to do a lot more testing to establish a diagnosis.

Providing Your Medical History

Here's a list of various questions that your doctor may ask you at your initial visit and the reasons why the questions are asked. These questions are posed mainly to ensure that no other diseases are present. Note that this list of questions is not meant to be exhaustive. *Part of any good medical history includes information about past surgeries, allergies and other illnesses, in addition to a family and social history.*

Question: Do you ever see blood in your urine?

Why the question is asked: Visible blood in the urine is uncommon in IC patients. Blood is seen more commonly in association with cancers of the urinary tract, kidney stone disease, or severe bladder infections.

Question: Do you ever get bladder infections? If yes, when was your last infection?

Why the question is asked: The symptoms of IC do not appear to be due to bladder infections; however, many IC patients have had bladder infections in the past. Some IC patients intermittently develop bladder infections that cause their symptoms to significantly worsen.

Question: Do you feel burning when you urinate?

Why the question is asked: Dysuria (burning when urinating) is commonly experienced with bladder infections and usually occurs only during urination. IC patients may have the sensation of "urethral" burning even when not urinating. (Urination takes place through the urethra.)

Question: Is there any personal or family history of kidney stones?

Why the question is asked: Stones in the urinary tract, particularly when in the lower portion of the ureter (the ureter is the tube that carries urine from the kidney to the bladder, see figure 1), may cause bladder symptoms. Occasionally, kidney stones can be hereditary.

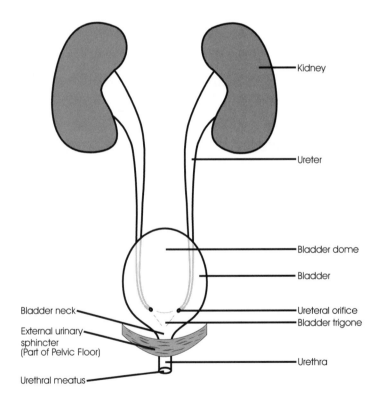

Figure 1. The urinary tract.

Question: Is there any history of sexually transmitted disease? Do you have any vaginal or urethral discharge?

Why the question is asked: Sexually transmitted diseases such as herpes, *Trichomonas*, yeast, gonorrhea, chancroid, and, occasionally, venereal warts can cause vaginal or pelvic discomfort.

Question: What was happening in your life around the time that your symptoms began? For example, were any of the following items present?

* Any surgeries? Pelvic radiation therapy?

* Any trauma?

* New medications?

* New laundry detergents?

* New bath soaps?

* New foods?

* New forms of contraception?

Why the question is asked: Any of these factors may cause either nerve and/or bladder injury or may cause local irritation to the vaginal walls.

Question: Do you leak urine?

Why the question is asked: There are several reasons urinary leakage can occur. Most of them have no relationship to IC. It's important to evaluate this problem, especially if the incontinence is related to severe urinary urgency. Urinary urgency resulting in incontinence may be due to problems as diverse as bladder cancer or neurological disease.

Now, here are some questions that your clinician may ask you to get a better understanding of the severity of your disease and to understand how it's affecting the quality of your life.

Question: How long have your symptoms been present?

Why the question is asked: IC is diagnosed today much earlier than in years past. When the patient exhibits typical symptoms and has failed a course or courses of antibiotics, the clinician usually considers the possibility of the disease. IC is much less likely to be found in a patient who has had symptoms for two weeks as opposed to a patient who has had two to three months of symptoms.

Question: Where is the exact location of your discomfort?

Why the question is asked: The location of discomfort gives important clues as to the source of pain. The discomfort associated with IC is usually in the middle of the abdomen, just above the pubic bone. The pain may radiate to the genitals, lower back, anus, or thighs.

Pain located to one side or another in the abdomen may be associated with other problems, such as a ruptured ovarian cyst or diverticulitis. It's been our observation that Hunner's ulcers associated with IC often cause pain related to their location on the bladder wall (left-sided Hunner's ulcer equals left-sided lower abdominal pain).

Question: Describe your discomfort.

Why the question is asked: Words often used by patients to describe their pain include the following: *stabbing, burning, twisting,* or *pressure.* The discomfort noted by those with IC varies in severity but generally the discomfort is chronic. Pain that is fleeting, lasts for several seconds or minutes and then disappears, is not characteristic of IC. That pain is more suggestive of a pelvic muscle spasm or of a gastrointestinal disorder.

Question: Describe the relationship of pain with urination.

Why the question is asked: The pain associated with interstitial cystitis often is significantly worsened with bladder filling. Bladder emptying usually causes a decrease in pelvic pain; albeit often only transiently. Although the absence of this symptom does not exclude a diagnosis of IC, the clinician must consider other causes of pelvic pain more seriously.

Question: Do your symptoms tend to change during the course of the day?

Why the question is asked: The symptoms of IC often change during the course of the day and vary from patient to patient. Often there is no obvious explanation for these fluctuations; however, factors such as physical activity (even just sitting or standing for long periods of time) or diet changes might influence symptoms.

Question: Does stress worsen your symptoms?

Why the question is asked: Although IC is not caused by stress, stress can be a major factor in the worsening of IC symptoms. It appears to particularly affect patients who have associated pelvic floor muscle spasm in addition to IC. The pelvic floor muscles normally support the pelvic organs (bladder, rectum, vagina, prostate, etc.) in place. These muscles normally relax when you urinate, have a bowel movement, or have sexual intercourse (see figure 2). Spasticity of these muscles commonly is seen in the IC patient and can give rise to symptoms of pelvic pain, urinary urgency and frequency. (This problem is discussed in detail in chapter 4, Medical Conditions Associated with Interstitial Cystitis.)

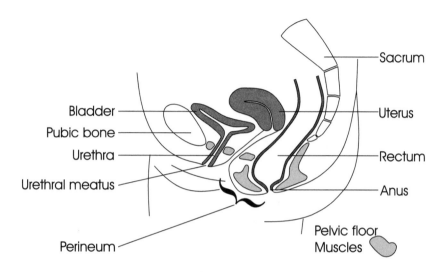

Figure 2. A side view of the female pelvis. Note the close association of the pelvic floor muscles to the bladder, urethra, vagina, and rectum.

Question: Do foods or beverages affect your symptoms?

Why the question is asked: Diet can have a profound effect on the symptoms of interstitial cystitis. Dietary changes frequently result in significant symptom improvement. (See chapter 10, Conservative Therapies for Interstitial Cystitis.)

Question: Have any activities or previous therapies helped to improve your symptoms?

Why the question is asked: This is a very important question for the clinician to ask. Patients with IC usually have seen more than one health care provider. Previous therapies may have been tried that might alter current treatment. For example:

1. A previous therapy might have been helpful but the side effects were intolerable to the patient. Sometimes changing the medication dose or the timing of the dose can help to

eliminate adverse reactions, thus making the drug usable again.

2. The history of previous therapies can guide the clinician away from forms of care that are unlikely to have any beneficial effect.

3. Patients often develop therapies of their own that help reduce symptoms. The clinician may be able to use that information to improve those therapies further or to suggest other forms of care to augment the initial therapy's effect.

Question: How many times do you awaken from sleep to void?

Why the question is asked: Interstitial cystitis usually causes patients to wake from sleep to urinate (a condition called *nocturia*). The answer to this question often correlates with the overall severity of disease. For example, voiding eight to twelve times per night suggests a very small bladder capacity. Patients who awaken this frequently at night commonly suffer from greater daytime fatigue and secondary problems such as depression and employment problems. Although IC can be diagnosed in the absence of nocturia, the diagnosis is less likely. In this instance, other pelvic problems such as pelvic floor muscle spasm are more likely to be the cause of the symptoms.

Question: Approximately how many times per day do you void?

Why the question is asked: The answer to this question is as important as the answer to the question regarding the nocturnal need to urinate. The answer provides information as to the impact that voiding has on the patient's daytime activities. For example, a patient who must void every twenty minutes obviously will have tremendous problems with a ninety-minute train commute to and from work. Questions regarding day and nighttime voiding are frequently followed by a request from the clinician to the patient to keep a "voiding diary." Patients are asked to record the time and the number of ounces voided during a twenty-four to forty-eight hour interval (see table 2.1). The voiding diary has several uses:

1. The diary establishes a "baseline" for a patient. The patient may be asked to record a diary and to do it again at a later date to see if a particular therapy, instituted between the two time points, had a beneficial effect. Over time and with appropriate therapy, one would hope to see less frequent and higher volume voids.

2. The diary helps the caregiver to make or exclude the diagnosis of IC. The typical patient with interstitial cystitis will have frequent and low volume voiding (one to four ounces). A patient who complains of urinary frequency every forty-five to sixty minutes but who voids 10–16 ounces per void is unlikely to have IC. Problems such as diabetes insipidus, diabetes mellitus, kidney disease, medication effect, or the compulsive intake of fluid (called "psychogenic polydipsia") must be considered.

Question: Do you use vaginal douches or vaginal deodorants?

Why the question is asked: Occasionally these products are related to an increase in vaginal discomfort, particularly in patients who have underlying hypersensitivity in that region. In some instances, these products can cause a "contact dermatitis" (local inflammation caused by contact with an allergy-causing substance). Also, the symptoms of vaginitis can be mistaken for bladder/urethral problems.

Question: Is intercourse painful?

Why the question is asked: Dyspareunia (painful intercourse) is noted in 50–75 percent of female IC patients. The pain is usually associated with penile pressure against the front portion of the vaginal wall. This is the region of the urethra and bladder. Other possible causes of dyspareunia include pelvic floor muscular tenderness or pain from the lining of the vagina itself.

Question: Does intercourse worsen your bladder symptoms?

Why the question is asked: Whether or not intercourse is painful, for the IC patient sexual intercourse can take a toll on bladder symptoms. Many IC patients complain that their pelvic discomfort and urinary frequency worsen several hours to one day after intercourse.

Question: Is ejaculation painful?

Why the question is asked: Ejaculation is a complex process that involves close communication between the nervous system, the muscles of the pelvic floor, the bladder, prostate, and seminal vesicles. Pain associated with ejaculation is a frequent complaint of the male IC patient and is probably related to one or a combination of these factors. In most instances, the pain seems to be related to severe spasm of the pelvic floor muscles. (See chapter 7, The Male with Interstitial Cystitis.)

Question: Do symptoms worsen during or one week prior to the menstrual period?

Table 2.1: Voiding Diary

IC Patient			Patient Less Likely to Have IC	
Time	**Ounces Voided**		**Time**	**Ounces Voided**
8:00 A.M.	1½		8:00 A.M.	10
8:25	3		9:30	6
9:00	3½		10:45	14
9:50	½		12:15 P.M.	8
10:30	4		1:45	4
11:15	2		3:00	6
11:30	2		4:30	10
12:45 P.M.	3½		6:10	6
2:00	4		6:30	12
2:15	1½		7:40	3
3:30	3		8:50	16
4:00	3		9:30	6
5:30	1½		10:45	8
7:00	2		11:45	4
7:45	2		1:30 A.M.	14
8:30	2½		4:15	9
10:00	3½		6:30	13
11:45	1		8:00	7
2:30 A.M.	4½			
4:50	3½			
6:30	2			
7:50	2½			
Total	56½		**Total**	156

Table 2.1 shows two 24-hour voiding diaries from two different patients. The left column depicts a patient with a relatively severe case of IC. Note the frequent small volume voids. (Keep in mind that this depicts the more severe form of disease. Many IC patients void higher volumes than depicted here.) The voiding pattern seen in the right column is unlikely to represent a patient with IC. Complaints of urinary frequency in this patient appear to be in large part due to very high voided volumes. Other problems such as diabetes must be considered for this patient.

Why the question is asked: Menstruation often worsens the symptoms of interstitial cystitis. Another complaint that is just as common is the worsening of symptoms seven to ten days prior to the menstrual flow. These patients usually report a significant reduction in symptoms during menstruation. The reason for these effects is unclear but it is likely (at least in part) that it relates to hormonal fluctuations and the release of inflammation-causing chemicals (such as prostaglandins) at these times.

Question: Any problems with constipation or irritable bowel syndrome?

Why the question is asked: Gastrointestinal disturbances may have a negative impact on the lower urinary tract in the patient with or without IC. In general, problems such as chronic constipation or irritable bowel syndrome intensify the symptoms of IC. To make matters worse, some medications that are otherwise useful in the management of IC can worsen these problems. The point here is that these gastrointestinal issues must be addressed by the treating clinician or in conjunction with a specialist (such as a gastroenterologist) to optimize therapy.

Question: Do you have a strong urine flow?

Why the question is asked: Women with IC often complain of a weak urine stream. Many factors can influence this problem. However, this situation is most often caused by the voiding of very low volumes (the bladder is not particularly efficient when contracting against very large or very small volumes) and/or abnormal simultaneous muscle contractions of the pelvic floor muscles (thus physically blocking the passage of urine). Men with IC may have these problems as well, but they too can be afflicted with the blockage of urine flow by the prostate gland.

Question: Is there any history of physical, sexual, or emotional abuse?

Why the question is asked: Occasionally, these types of stresses have been found to be associated with pelvic and/or vaginal pain. This problem appears to arise from muscle spasm in these regions.

What to Expect During Your Physical Examination

The main reason for the physical examination is to identify any other medical problems that could cause similar symptoms to IC. Your abdomen is examined for the presence of masses, hernias, or the location and nature of any pain that is present. Mild abdominal fullness may be seen and is most commonly associated with chronic constipation. Most often, when pain is present, it will be located in your abdomen just above the pubic bone. In women, the pelvic examination can give many clues to suggest IC and/or other medical problems.

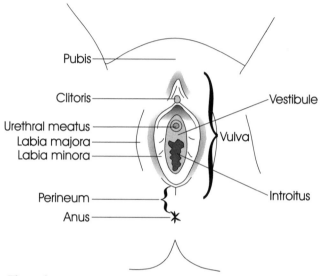

Figure 3. The vulva.

The external genital region (vulva) (see figure 3) and vagina are inspected. The major factors that are evaluated include:

The presence of diseased tissue in this area

* The area is inspected for *atrophic changes* (tissue that is thin and pale in appearance). Vaginal wall atrophy often occurs after menopause and is due to loss of estrogen. It can be associated with extra sensitivity and/or itching in that area. Atrophy of the vaginal wall can also encourage the development of urinary tract infections.

* The vaginal wall and vulva are inspected for the lesions of herpes, venereal warts (also called *condyloma*), lichen sclerosis, psoriasis, and eczema.

The presence of vaginal discharge

Vaginal discharge is a normal finding; however, certain qualities of the discharge may indicate infectious processes. For example:

* *Yeast infection:* Whitish, creamy, odorless discharge.

* *Trichomonas infection:* Discharge may be frothy and green to yellowish in appearance. The infection can be associated with small bleeding points on the cervix and vagina. This organism can be sexually transmitted.

* *Bacterial vaginosis:* Foul smelling (fishy odor) discharge that is usually thin and clear to grayish-yellow in appearance. The infection is caused by anerobic organisms (organisms that don't need oxygen to grow and multiply).

The presence of vulvar pain

The specific site of your pain should be identified. Pain or swelling around the urethra can be caused by infected glands or cysts in this region. The examiner may press into different areas of the vagina and vulva to better determine the source of pain. The urethra is inspected by running a finger along the front portion of the vaginal wall. A lump in this area or discharge from the urethra is suggestive of an urethral diverticulum, which is an abnormal, small "pouch" that protrudes from the urethra that can become infected (see figure 4).

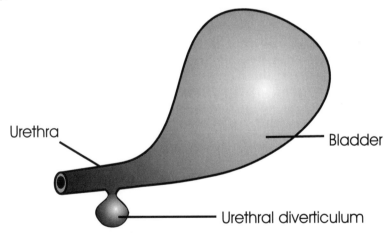

Figure 4. A urethral diverticulum is a small pouch that originates from the lining of the urethra. It is often associated with dribbling after urination. This occurs due to urine filling this sac during urination. The urine that collects in the diverticulum then slowly drains *after* urination has been completed. Other problems associated with the urethral diverticulum include recurrent urinary tract infections, pain with sexual intercourse, and pain with urination. If the clinician suspects that a urethral diverticulum exists, special x-ray tests usually are performed for further evaluation.

Examination then proceeds deeper into the vagina. Pelvic organs such as the uterus, cervix, and ovaries are examined. Deep tenderness along the front portion of the vagina suggests that the pain is located in the lower portion of the bladder. At this time, the clinician may inspect for the presence of pelvic floor muscle tenderness.

The pelvic floor muscles support your pelvic organs and are important in maintaining your ability to hold urine and stool as well as having sexual relations. Pelvic floor muscle spasticity is often found in IC patients, and accounts for pain when mild pressure is applied to the deep vaginal sidewalls. The normal consistency of this region is soft; however, many patients with pelvic floor muscle spasm are found to have "tight" muscle bands, similar in feel to a taut violin bowstring. A rectal examination may be performed to assure that no masses are present. The rectal examination can also detect the presence of muscle tenderness.

You might be asked to "bear down" or to cough. This often unmasks the presence of a *cystocoele*—a "dropped" bladder. (The bladder can be seen protruding into the vagina.) (See figure 5.)

Cystocoeles and Rectocoeles

Cystocoeles are rarely associated with pelvic or vaginal discomfort unless they are relatively large. In some instances, they can be the cause of *urinary incontinence* (uncontrolled loss of urine) or *urinary retention* (inability to completely empty the bladder). A *rectocoele* may also be found during this part of the examination. In this instance, the rectum bulges into the vagina in much the same way that the bladder can bulge from the front of the vagina. A rectocoele is frequently associated with chronic constipation since the stool tends to collect in the "bulge" rather than moving easily across the anus.

Examination of Males

A male with suspected IC needs a detailed examination of his genitalia and rectum. The penis is inspected for the presence of skin lesions or discharge. Patients with IC often complain of scrotal or testicular discomfort. The skin of the scrotum is examined for evidence of rashes or other lesions. The testicle and spermatic cord (a cord-like structure that supplies the testicles with blood and also transports sperm through the vas deferens) are also examined for masses or specific sites of tenderness.

Pain sensed by the patient with IC in this region is usually "referred" pain. This means that the pain actually originates from

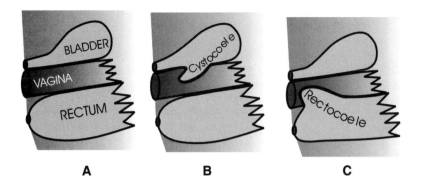

Figure 5. Problems that can occur due to "defects" in the pelvic floor. A. Normal anatomy. B. Cystocoele or the "dropped bladder." In this instance, the bladder is pushing out into the vaginal cavity. A cystocoele can be associated with urinary leakage, the inability to empty the bladder completely (you can see how urine might collect in this sac), or with pelvic/vaginal discomfort. In some instances, the cystocoele can be so large that it extends outside the vagina. C. A rectocoele is essentially the same problem as the cystocoele; however in this case, it's the rectum that is pushing into the vagina. Many patients have *both* a cystocoele and rectocoele.

another site (such as the bladder, prostate, or pelvic floor muscles); however, due to complex neurological channels, the pain is perceived at a different site. As a consequence of this phenomenon, the patient may complain of constant testicular pain but examination of the testicle is unremarkable.

The rectal examination is performed to exclude the presence of rectal masses or prostate nodules. Cancers of these organs rarely produce symptoms until a relatively advanced stage. The prostate is also examined for tenderness. Pressing on the prostate at this time may produce prostatic secretions (seen at the tip of the penis) that can be examined microscopically and sent to a laboratory for a culture. The pelvic floor muscles may also be examined at this time for tenderness. (See also chapter 7, The Male with Interstitial Cystitis.)

Tests Used to Diagnose Interstitial Cystitis

You'll see a lot of tests mentioned in this section. Most of the testing is used to exclude other diseases that may have similar symptoms and physical findings as IC. But it's quite unlikely that you'll be subjected to every test mentioned here. The choice of testing is based upon the clinician's suspicion of what might be causing your problem.

The Urinalysis

The urinalysis is a standard test to identify abnormalities in the urine. These abnormalities can suggest the presence of various diseases. Urinalysis can be divided into two parts: the dipstick and microscopic exams.

The Dipstick Exam

Using this quickly performed test, the urine is examined for the presence and quantity of glucose, ketones, pH, and blood. Glucose in the urine is important to note because it suggests that diabetes might be present (diabetes mellitus is a common cause of frequent urination). Blood in the urine is another very important finding. Blood detected in the urine can come from anywhere in the urinary tract, from the kidneys to the urethra. When blood is found in the absence of urinary tract infection, further evaluation may be indicated to exclude the existence of tumors, urinary tract stone disease, etc.

The detection of a urinary tract infection can often be accomplished with the use of nitrite and leukocyte esterase testing, both of which are part of some dipstick evaluations. *Nitrite testing* detects the presence of bacteria; however, a few types of bacteria fail to register positive on this evaluation. Also, low counts of bacteria may not be detected by this method. *Leukocyte esterase testing* determines the presence of white blood cells (pus cells) in the urine. These cells are identified in most infections. When used together, nitrite and leukocyte esterase testing are about 85 percent accurate in the diagnosis of a urinary tract infection.

The Microscopic Exam

A microscopic examination is very helpful to confirm the results of a dipstick examination and offers some information that the dipstick cannot provide. The microscopic examination is used to directly identify the presence of bacteria, white blood cells, red blood cells, and other abnormalities such as crystals in the urine.

The Urine Culture and Sensitivity

Taking a urine culture provides a more sensitive method to determine the presence of a urinary tract infection and should be used in conjunction with a urinalysis. Additionally, sensitivity testing determines which antibiotics have the best chance of eradicating the offending bacteria. When a bacterium has been identified by a laboratory, a "colony count" is reported. This number tells the clinician the concentration of bacteria in the specimen. Many IC patients experience a worsening of their symptoms when low numbers of organisms are present. Unfortunately, many laboratories do not report low counts of bacteria, assuming that they are not clinically significant or are contaminants. Often, special arrangements are necessary between the clinician and the laboratory to obtain these results.

Urine Cytology

In some instances, bladder cancer can cause symptoms of urgency and frequency of urination. The urine cytology exam evaluates cells that are shed into the urine. The specimen is evaluated by a cytopathologist who determines whether the cells look cancerous or noncancerous. The test is fairly accurate for high-grade (very aggressive, tending to spread quickly) tumors of the urinary tract but less so for low-grade (less aggressive, slow-growing) tumors.

Special Cultures

In situations where a high degree of suspicion exists, testing for sexually transmitted diseases (for example, chlamydia, gonorrhea, herpes, and syphilis) may be performed. Testing can be accomplished using cultures or special molecular biological diagnostic techniques. Tuberculosis is an infectious disease that can affect the bladder and isn't detected in standard cultures. The finding of unexplained pus in the urine or a high rate of tuberculosis in the community may warrant specific testing for tuberculosis.

The Pelvic Ultrasound Exam

Although most major abnormalities within the pelvis can be detected upon a pelvic exam, the pelvic ultrasound has been helpful in picking up subtle abnormalities of the gynecological organs such as ovarian cystic disease and uterine fibroids. The pelvic ultrasound is also helpful in the identification of fluid collections in the pelvis, a finding commonly seen with infections. This can be a tough test for the IC patient since the standard method of pelvic ultrasonography requires a full bladder. One alternative to this technique is to use a vaginal ultrasound probe for the exam. The bladder doesn't need to be distended in this instance, but manipulation during the procedure can temporarily worsen IC symptoms.

The IVP (Intravenous Pyelogram)

Stones in the lower ureter can cause urgency and frequency of urination. This usually occurs prior to the passage of the stone into the bladder and is often accompanied by blood in the urine. Occasionally, the blood can be seen by the naked eye but, in most instances, it can be seen only under the microscope. The IVP is an x-ray examination of the urinary tract. An iodine-based contrast solution is administered intravenously. The medication is concentrated in the kidney and is passed in the urine. The contrast solution in the urinary tract allows the kidneys, ureters, and bladder to be seen with x-rays.

The patient may experience a warm sensation after injection of the contrast solution. Occasionally, nausea can occur. An allergic reaction to the solution can also occur and in rare instances can be life-threatening. Patients with an allergy to iodine (such as in shellfish) or a history of asthma appear to have a higher rate of adverse reaction and are, therefore, usually premedicated with an antihistamine and/or a steroid. These patients also are given a contrast solution with a decreased potential for allergic reaction ("nonionic contrast"). IC patients do not seem to have a higher rate of adverse reactions than the general population.

Urodynamic Evaluation

Urodynamic evaluation provides information regarding the *function* of the lower urinary tract and comprises the following tests:

The Uroflow Exam

The uroflow exam is a graphical depiction of the patient's urine flow rate. The parameters assessed include the volume voided, the peak flow rate (the fastest speed that the urine comes out of the body when voiding), and the average flow rate. (By constantly monitoring the speed with which urine leaves the body, a computer can calculate average flow rate.) The uroflow exam can help the clinician to determine the presence of blockages in the passage of urine or abnormal behavior of the bladder. The test is often performed along with a cystometrogram (see below) to obtain the most accurate results. The test is performed by having you void into a specially designed commode. The computer does the rest of the work. The most common problem encountered when testing the IC patient (and many non-IC patients as well) is the inability to void in the office setting.

The Post-Void Volume Assessment (PVR)

The act of urination normally releases all the urine that collected in the bladder. Abnormal bladder function or blockages to the flow of urine from the bladder (such as the prostate, scar tissue, or abnormal tightening of the pelvic floor muscles) may result in the retention of some urine. In instances where a great deal of urine is left in the bladder, the clinician can feel bladder fullness when pressing upon the lower abdomen. Alternatively, a catheter can be placed into the bladder in order to measure the residual urine. Most recently, special ultrasound units have been developed to determine the *post-void residual* urine volume (PVR) in the office setting. This has been a particularly helpful development for the IC patient, many of whom have significant discomfort with catheter insertion. The PVR is important for diagnosis because high residual volumes usually indicate some functional or anatomical problem in the lower urinary tract.

The Cystometrogram (CMG)

The cystometrogram is a test of bladder function. It's often used to identify the cause of urinary incontinence or the inability to urinate. The cystometrogram can also give clues to the sensitivity of the bladder surface and how easily the bladder stretches when being filled.

A skinny catheter is placed into the urethra and advanced into the bladder. The bladder is then slowly filled with sterile water while the patient is monitored and asked frequent questions. Patients are asked at what time they first sense some bladder filling and at what time they sense the first urge to void. They are asked to state when they feel that they have to urinate. Finally, the patient is asked to urinate. All this time a computer is measuring the pressures that are generated by the bladder.

Usually, IC patients are found to have low volumes of fluid in their bladders when they first sense fullness. The *bladder capacity* (how much the bladder can hold) of most IC patients is also pretty low.

There exists some controversy regarding the role of the cystometrogram in evaluating the IC patient. Many physicians perform this test on all patients. They feel that the information generated by this test helps them to better understand the severity of disease and to make predictions of how a given patient will respond to therapy. Others (including those at our Center) generally reserve this testing for select patients, primarily those who don't empty their bladders effectively or those who have associated urinary incontinence.

Colposcopy

Colposcopy is usually performed to identify very small lesions of the vaginal wall. The *colposcope* is essentially a very strong magnifying glass. Gynecologists or gynecological nurse practitioners usually perform colposcopy. The procedure is usually performed because of an abnormal PAP smear. This is not a routine procedure in the evaluation of the IC patient; however, it may be helpful in evaluating the presence of associated vaginal pain.

Laparoscopy

Laparoscopy is a surgical procedure that allows inspection of the abdominal cavity without requiring a big incision. It is carried out by introducing a gas (carbon dioxide) into the abdominal cavity through a special needle. A telescope, called a *laparoscope*, is then introduced into the abdomen through an inconspicuous, small incision in the navel. The abdominal contents and pelvic organs can then be inspected. By inserting other skinny "ports" at other sites in the abdomen, instruments can be introduced and surgery can be performed. Laparoscopy is another procedure that is not routinely used in evaluating the IC patient. In the patient with chronic pelvic pain, its most common use is in the diagnosis of endometriosis or ovarian problems.

Cystoscopy

Cystoscopy is a common urological procedure that allows a magnified inspection of the bladder and urethra. Cystoscopy is usually carried out in the office setting, however; it also can be performed in the operating room in those cases where urethral pain is too severe.

Two forms of cystoscopy exist: rigid and flexible. Rigid cystoscopy employs a metal instrument whereas flexible cystoscopy uses a small caliber instrument that is very similar to a standard soft urethral catheter. The flexible cystoscope is made of flexible plastic and has a tip that can move, thereby allowing excellent inspection of all surfaces. As you can imagine, most IC patients (in fact, almost *all* patients—particularly men) prefer flexible office cystoscopy to the rigid type.

The purpose of cystoscopy is to identify abnormalities of the urethra and/or bladder surface. For example, examination of the urethra might reveal inflammatory changes, scar tissue (*stricture* disease), or even cancer. In the male patient, the prostatic urethra (the region of the urethra that passes through the prostate gland) is evaluated to determine how big the prostate is or to check for the presence of inflammation. Fluid, usually sterile water, is used to distend the bladder so that the surface can be inspected for irregularities. The bladder capacity can be grossly assessed by the amount of fluid that can be introduced—keeping in mind that bladder filling during cystoscopy is rather rapid and that this can cause the early sensation of filling and the need to urinate. Patches of redness may indicate inflammation (Hunner's ulcer) or flat cancers (*carcinoma in situ*). Bladder cancers, bladder stones, or congenital abnormalities of the bladder or lower ureter can be seen. Additionally, the two regions where urine enters the bladder can be examined (the ureteral orifices). Urine can normally be seen "jetting" from these holes. Finally, processes such as fibroid disease of the uterus can be indirectly noted by extrinsic compression of the bladder wall.

Inserting a cystoscope into the bladder is similar to having a urethral catheter placed. The procedure is described in chapter 6, Medications Introduced into the Bladder.

Cystoscopy performed in the office has a limited role in the diagnosis of interstitial cystitis since most patients have no abnormal findings. The only exception to this statement relates to the small number of patients (less than 10 percent of all IC patients) who have patchy areas of surface redness associated with severe inflammation (Hunner's ulcers). These abnormal regions of the bladder surface first require biopsy to exclude the possibility of cancer. Areas of redness and/or scarring from previous biopsy sites are often mistaken for Hunner's ulcers. On occasion, insertion of the cystoscope causes a region of bladder wall irritation that may also be misinterpreted as a Hunner's patch. In summary, the most important reason to perform cystoscopy is to exclude other disease processes that can cause similar symptoms to IC.

Cystoscopy with Hydrodistention

Cystoscopy with hydrodistention of the bladder is considered to be the "gold standard" technique to *aid* in diagnosing interstitial cystitis. There is a stress on the word *aid* here because a diagnosis of IC should never be based on the results of this test alone. The procedure is performed by first placing the patient under anesthesia (usually general or spinal anesthesia). A cystoscopic examination is carried out. Irregularities of the bladder wall are sought. A Hunner's ulcer (or patch) might be identified at this time. The bladder is then distended to fairly high pressures using the fluid running through the cystoscope.

The IC bladder is very sensitive and commonly develops superficial surface tears during the filling procedure. These regions heal rapidly. Full thickness bladder tears are extremely rare events seen only in the most severe cases of IC.

Once the bladder achieves its maximum filling pressure, the fluid is left in place from two to eight minutes. Then the fluid is released into a measuring container and the volume is recorded as the *anesthetic bladder capacity*. This volume can be very helpful in evaluating an IC patient.

The normal adult's bladder capacity under anesthesia generally ranges from 800–1,200 cc; however, the average capacity of most IC patients is approximately 600–700 cc. Does this mean that if a patient has an anesthetic bladder capacity of 1,100 cc, that the patient doesn't have IC? Absolutely not, but it does make the clinician suspect other causes for symptoms. The anesthetic bladder capacity also gives the clinician some idea of disease severity and even of the prospects for recovery. It will probably be more difficult to manage a patient with a bladder capacity of 200 cc as opposed to a patient with a 700 cc capacity.

The bladder is then slowly filled again and inspected for the presence of *glomerulations*. These are small bleeding points on the bladder surface which are often seen in patients with IC. Clinicians used to rely on the presence of these bleeding points to make a diagnosis of IC. Recent observations, however, demonstrate that the presence of glomerulations doesn't always correlate with a diagnosis of IC. Yes, they're more commonly seen in IC, but they may be present in many other bladder diseases and may even be present in patients without bladder disease. Furthermore, many patients with the most severe form of IC, those with scarred, shrunken bladders, have no glomerulations at all.

The Bladder Biopsy

Many clinicians will obtain a bladder biopsy at the same time a bladder hydrodistention is performed. Here, a *biopsy forceps* is advanced through the cystoscope. The bladder wall is grasped and a tiny piece of tissue is removed (roughly the size of this dot ●). This tissue is sent for microscopic evaluation. Often, special staining techniques are used when looking for specific types of inflammation.

One form of inflammation that has been seen in many IC patients involves the presence of many *mast* cells and has been termed *detrusor (bladder) mastocytosis*. The mast cell is a specific type of cell that causes inflammation. It does this by secreting substances such as histamine, prostaglandins, and leukotrienes—all chemicals that stimulate the inflammatory process. The biopsies of most patients with IC demonstrate mild to moderate inflammation. Patients with the classical form of IC (severe disease) often have more bladder inflammation and *fibrosis* (scarring) of the bladder wall.

The Potassium Sensitivity Test

The potassium sensitivity test (PST) is a relatively recent addition to diagnostic evaluation. The concept here is that many patients with IC have an abnormality of the bladder surface that allows small, noxious substances like potassium and urea to be absorbed. These molecules can stimulate nerves, thereby causing discomfort, and they may also cause inflammation in the bladder wall.

The test is performed in three steps. First, a thin catheter is introduced into the bladder. Sterile water is then introduced and the patient is asked if any pain results. This establishes a *baseline* of pain with just bladder filling. The patient then urinates and the same volume of a potassium chloride solution is instilled. An increase in pain by 2 on a 0–5 pain scale (5 being severe pain) suggests that IC is present. The potassium chloride solution is then removed via the catheter. For those patients who experience continued pain after the procedure is over, most clinicians will introduce an anesthetic solution into the bladder.

At the time of this writing, there exists some controversy over which is the best testing to perform in evaluating the IC patient, hydrodistention or PST. Here are some pros and cons of each procedure.

Hydrodistention Test

Advantages include the following:

* The bladder can be inspected for evidence of tumors or inflammation.

* If desired, a bladder biopsy can be obtained.

* The anesthetic bladder capacity can be determined. This information is helpful for diagnosis and prognosis and may help guide therapy. For example, a patient with a very small bladder capacity might benefit with a bladder retraining

protocol. (See chapter 10, Conservative Therapies for Interstitial Cystitis.)

* The procedure may improve symptoms. 30–60% of IC patients will have symptom improvement from the procedure; however, symptom worsening should be expected to occur for 2–3 weeks immediately after the procedure.

Disadvantages include the following:

* The procedure must be performed under anesthesia.

* There are some operative risks, albeit they are very low.

* Only urologists and specially trained gynecologists ("urogynecologists") are capable of performing cystoscopy.

Potassium Sensitivity Test (PST)

Advantages include the following:

* The procedure is performed on an outpatient basis with no associated operative risks.

* PST is generally associated with a more rapid patient recovery time; however, the test may cause a flare-up of symptoms in some patients.

* PST can be performed by nonurologists.

Disadvantages include the following:

* Does not allow inspection of the bladder wall. Therefore, the physician may advise an office cystoscopy.

* Does not allow biopsy.

* Patients may experience severe pain in the office during and after the procedure. Usually this problem can be managed by the instillation of an anesthetic into the bladder at the end of the procedure.

* Positive testing may occur in patients with other bladder disorders.

* Negative results may occur in an IC patient who is receiving therapy for IC.

Probably the most important question regarding these procedures is, which is the best one to help make the diagnosis of IC? The answer is a bit complicated. First, notice that I stated *"to help* make the diagnosis." That's because, as mentioned earlier in this chapter, the diagnosis is made by putting *all* the clinical information together.

The clinician cannot make the diagnosis of IC solely on the basis of either of these two tests. To really drive this point home, a recent study (Teichman and B. J. Neilsen-Omeis 1999) evaluated 38 IC patients and subjected them to PST. Twenty-three patients were positive (increased pain with potassium chloride instillation) and 15 patients were negative. Therefore, if we were to use only the results of the PST to establish a diagnosis of IC, 15 out of 38 patients in this study would never have been diagnosed, and would probably not have received therapy.

On the other hand, it is likely there are many patients who will have a significant response to the PST and have relatively unremarkable findings upon bladder hydrodistention. So, what does all of this mean? It means that neither test is perfect but each may help the physician arrive at the diagnosis. The form of testing that is offered to the patient depends upon the individual physician's comfort with these procedures and their interpretation of the literature. We have not made use of the potassium sensitivity test due to the disadvantages described above, particularly the significant discomfort that is created for some patients.

Other Tests That May Be Useful to Diagnose IC

Let's face it. The thought of going through a procedure that needs to be performed in the operating room or one that causes your bladder to burn is not a particularly joyful notion. For this reason, we're constantly looking for ways to reach a diagnosis with less attendant "body trauma." Here are some new methods of evaluation, some being used right now, but most still under investigation.

Response to Anesthetic Instillation

We have been using this simple technique for the past several years. It is helpful in assessing whether the bladder is the source of pelvic discomfort. An anesthetic solution containing a long- and short-acting anesthetic (bupivacaine/lidocaine) is introduced into the bladder and held for about twenty minutes. *Improvement* in pelvic discomfort shortly after administration suggests that the patient's pain originates from the bladder (hence, bladder oversensitivity). Just as with the potassium sensitivity test, this evaluation cannot assure that no other bladder problems are present (such as infection or tumors).

We have reviewed 28 patients with IC and pelvic pain. Twenty patients had decreased pain after instillation. The advantage here is that patients usually leave the office quite comfortable. In some cases, improvement in symptoms can last for one to two weeks. In rare cases, patients have had a temporary symptom flare when the anesthetic effect wore off.

Urine "Markers" for Diagnosis of Interstitial Cystitis

Of course, the best test possible to diagnose interstitial cystitis would be one that is completely painless and simple to perform. That issue has led investigators to search for a "marker" of interstitial cystitis in the urine. Several investigators have identified changes in the urine of IC patients. These changes might be helpful in making the diagnosis of IC in the future. Some studies completed over the past eight years include the following:

Hurst, Parsons, Roy, and Young (1993) have shown that complex molecules called glycosaminoglycans are found in low concentration in the urine of most IC patients when compared to people without IC.

Erickson, Sheykhnazari, Ordille, and Bhavanandan (1998) found increased amounts of hyaluronic acid in the urine of IC patients. This finding is particularly interesting since hyaluronic acid is normally found beneath the bladder surface. To find this chemical in the urine suggests that the bladder wall in IC patients is "leaky." This leakiness may be one of the factors that cause the disease (see chapter 3, What Causes Interstitial Cystitis?). This group (1996) also found decreased levels of urinary epitectin (also called MUC-1 glycoprotein) in the urine of IC patients.

Another well-studied potential marker for interstitial cystitis is GP51. This is a large molecule that is normally present on the bladder's surface and in the urine. We (Moskowitz, Shupp-Byrne, Callahan, Parsons, Valderrama, and Moldwin 1994) initially demonstrated GP51 levels to be lower in the bladder biopsies of most IC patients. Recently, the same findings (low GP51 levels) have been found in the urine of IC patients (Shupp-Byrne, Sedor, Estojak, Fitzpatrick et al. 1999).

Keay, Zhang, Hise, Hebel, et al. (1998) have shown that the urine of IC patients can inhibit the growth of bladder cells when cultured in a laboratory setting.

This is not meant to be an exhaustive list of studies hoping to find a "marker" for IC. Rather, it should demonstrate to the reader that this is an area of great interest to researchers. At the time of this writing, these tests are not used routinely in the diagnosis of IC and are not available in any clinical laboratory.

The NIDDK Criteria for Interstitial Cystitis

As has been mentioned, the diagnosis of interstitial cystitis is made on the basis of excluding other diseases *and* establishing that the bladder is overly sensitive. The diagnosis is fairly easy to make in patients with severe symptoms; however, clinicians sometimes disagree on the diagnosis in the patient with mild symptoms. This difference in patient evaluation and diagnosis can pose a problem when evaluating research studies from one institution to another.

For example, suppose Institution A wants to investigate a new medication to decrease patient symptoms. Institution A enrolls only patients into the study who urinate more than four times per night and more than thirty times during the day. Institution B's criteria for patient enrollment are far less rigorous. Patients in their study need only to urinate more than nine times per day and the lack of nighttime urinary frequency doesn't exclude the diagnosis of IC. Most clinicians would consider the symptom criteria established by Institution A to be a bit too rigorous.

Conversely, the criteria to establish a diagnosis of interstitial cystitis by Institution B might be considered by some clinicians to be rather loose. Each group considers the other group's diagnosis of interstitial cystitis invalid, thereby bringing medical progress to a dead halt. In order to limit this problem, the National Institutes of Diabetes, Digestive, and Kidney Diseases (NIDDK), a branch of the National Institutes of Health, formed a consensus panel in 1987 and 1988. Criteria were established for the diagnosis of IC to be used in *research studies* (see table 2.2). Please keep in mind that these criteria were established to standardize scientific studies. These criteria select patients with moderate to severe symptoms. They were *not* established to be used in the routine diagnosis of IC. If used in that capacity, approximately 60 percent of IC patients will not be diagnosed and therefore not receive appropriate treatment (Hanno, Landis, Matthews-Cook, Kusek, et al. 1999).

Table 2.2: NIDDK Criteria for the Diagnosis of Interstitial Cystitis

Required Findings:

Hunner's ulcer or diffuse glomerulations (small bleeding points on the bladder surface seen after hydrodistention of the bladder)

and

Pain associated with the bladder or urinary urgency

Automatic Exclusions:

Less than 18 years of age

Duration of symptoms less than 9 months

Urinary frequency of less than 8 times per day

Absence of nocturia (nighttime urination)

Benign or malignant bladder tumors

Radiation cystitis (irritation of the bladder from radiation therapy)

Tuberculous cystitis (infection of the bladder from tuberculosis)

Bacterial cystitis (the common urinary tract infection) or prostatitis (prostate infection)

Vaginitis

Cyclophosphamide cystitis (inflammation of the bladder which can occur after cyclophosphamide chemotherapy)

Urethral diverticulum (an anatomical abnormality of the urethra which can cause urine dribbling, recurrent urinary tract infections, burning with urination, etc.)

Uterine, cervical, vaginal, or urethral cancer

Active herpes

Bladder or lower ureteral calculi (stones in the bladder or lower portion of the tubes which transport urine from the kidneys to the bladder)

Symptoms relieved by antibiotics, urinary antiseptics, urinary analgesics, anticholinergics (bladder muscle relaxants), or antispasmotics (muscle relaxants like Valium or Robaxin)

Involuntary bladder contractions (see evaluation of the IC patient-urodynamics)

Bladder capacity less than 350 cc while awake

Chapter **3**

What Causes Interstitial Cystitis?

Theories abound regarding the cause of interstitial cystitis (IC) but we still don't have a definitive answer. Most investigators agree that there may be several causes for the development of symptoms. This may be why patient responses to therapy vary so widely. Over the past several years, many abnormalities of the "IC bladder" have been identified which probably have a significant impact on patient complaints. Let's review some of these abnormalities.

Abnormalities of the Bladder's Surface

Abnormalities of the bladder's surface have been seen in most IC patients. In the normal setting, the bladder lining is quite amazing. It's able to hold urine, a rather noxious solution, and dramatically expand without leaking any toxins back into the body. The bladder surface accomplishes this task admirably, but sometimes problems do occur.

Bladder Surface Mucin

The bladder's surface secretes a complex material, termed bladder surface mucin or bladder slime. The latter name comes from the slimy consistency of this layer. Bladder surface mucin appears to serve a very important role in preventing bacteria from adhering to the underlying bladder wall (the urothelial surface). Thus, this layer helps to prevent bladder infections. Bladder surface mucin also seems to prevent the absorption of the caustic components of urine into the deeper layers of the bladder wall. If "leakage" of this sort were to occur, its direct effect upon the nerves of the bladder would be like pouring salt into an open wound! The appearance of urine in a location where it's not supposed to be also could directly stimulate inflammation of the bladder wall.

In support of this theory, Drs. Lilly and Parsons (1990) at UCLA– San Diego have demonstrated increased absorption of small molecules in the bladder walls of IC patients as compared to non-IC patients. Chemical treatment to remove bladder surface mucin placed into the bladders of normal volunteers caused many of the symptoms of IC.

Using electron microscopy, no changes in the bladder surface have been seen in IC patients (Dixon, Holm-Bentzen, Gilpin, Gosling, et al. 1986); however, biochemical studies of the bladder's surface have revealed qualitative changes (Moskowitz, Shupp-Byrne, Callahan, Parsons, Valderrama, and Moldwin 1994). For example, GP51, a large molecule that is normally secreted by the bladder's lining, is found in decreased amounts on the bladder surface of most IC patients when compared to people without IC. Furthermore, GP51 is found in reduced amounts in the urine of most IC patients (see "Urine Markers for Diagnosis of Interstitial Cystitis" in chapter 2).

Changes in the Nerves of IC Patients

Alterations of the nerves within the wall of the bladder have been noted in IC patients. Some investigators have seen increased numbers of pain-carrying nerves, called C-fibers, in bladder biopsies from IC patients (Pang, Marchand, Sant, Kream, et al. 1993). These fibers carry and can release a chemical called Substance P. Substance P has the ability to transmit pain information in the nervous system and has been shown to stimulate inflammation. Our laboratory has recently shown heightened levels of Substance P in the urine of IC patients. Interestingly, the substance P levels go up when patients are in "flare" but go down when patients have few symptoms (Chen, Varghese, Lehrer, Tillem, Moldwin, and Kushner 1999).

Abnormalities of the Bladder's Blood Supply

For the survival of all cells in our bodies, oxygen is a basic requirement. One of the major roles of the bloodstream is to transport oxygen to these cells. Complete oxygen deprivation for even short periods of time can lead to cell death. Partial oxygen deprivation often leads to abnormalities in cell behavior and to pain. Such a situation exists in a disease called reflex sympathetic dystrophy (RSD).

In RSD, the sympathetic nervous system, that part of our nervous system that is responsible for functions such as increasing heart rate and raising blood pressure, begins to work in an uncontrolled fashion. It causes blood vessels to constrict and thereby can prevent blood from reaching various parts of the body. Most typically, the changes of RSD are seen in the extremities, where because of the lack of blood flow, pain begins. The constant decrease in blood flow can result in atrophy (wasting away) of the limb. It's thought that this same process might be taking place in patients with the classical form of IC, the form associated with bladder scarring.

Doctors Irwin and Galloway (1993) were the first to report a relative lack of blood flow in the bladders' of IC patients when compared to non-IC patients during bladder filling. Pontari, Hanno, and Ruggieri (1999) recently demonstrated similar findings but could not relate the changes in blood flow to the severity of symptoms. Abnormalities in bladder blood flow suggest that medications like nifedipine (see chapter 5, Oral Medications) that have been used to treat RSD might help some IC patients.

Undiagnosed Microorganisms

The role of microorganisms in the IC patient has been controversial since the original description of the disease. After all, the symptoms of IC sure sound very much like those of a urinary tract infection—but, of course, no infection is routinely detected. Prior to their diagnosis, many IC patients have had one or more unsuccessful courses of antibiotics (even in the face of normal urinalyses and cultures). This frequent scenario has led most clinicians to discard the idea that the disease is related to infection. Some even speculated that antibiotics might be the cause the disease (Holm-Bentzen, Nordling, and Hald 1990). Elgavish, Pattanaik, Lloyd, and Reed (1994, 1997) noted that many IC patients have had bladder infections in the past. They suggested that perhaps the infection went away but the bladder insult remained.

Still, many patients and researchers have been concerned that we've been missing some causative organism that is present in low numbers in the bladder that is resistant to standard antibiotic therapy. They point out similarities between IC and bladder infections. For example, just like most urinary tract infections, many IC patients report a rather rapid onset of symptoms. And just like most urinary tract infections, IC is much more common in women. Furthermore, lots of patients with interstitial cystitis have had documented bladder infections in the past.

In recent years there was an unrelated but very interesting discovery made that shocked the medical community. Researchers found that stomach ulcer disease can actually be caused by an unusual infectious organism (Helicobacter pylori), a concept that had been shrugged off by many clinicians as impossible for many years. Even better, these ulcers can be healed with appropriate antibiotic therapy. This last finding and the similarities between IC and bladder infections have fueled continued interest in the role that microorganisms might play in IC.

Research in this field is not easy. Here are some of the problems that arise when studies are conducted:

1. Probably the biggest problem faced by investigators is that different people respond in different ways to microorganisms. Many people have loads of bacteria in their bladder along with pus, but they have absolutely no symptoms of a bladder infection. This is called asymptomatic bacteriuria and it is treated with antibiotics only in special circumstances. Conversely, some patients develop terrible symptoms of pelvic pain, burning with urination, urinary urgency and frequency with such small numbers of bacteria that standard urine cultures don't identify the organism. So it's not only important to identify that an organism is present—any investigation must also show that eradication of the organism results in symptom improvement. Failure to link these two issues in the IC patient has been the major limitation of studies to date.

2. Urine cultures taken from patients can be contaminated by microorganisms found in the vagina or on the outside of the urethra. In routine practice, when contamination of the urine is an issue, the clinician might wish to catheterize the patient in order to avoid extraneous germs. Unfortunately, even placing a catheter into the urethra can push very small numbers of bacteria from the outside of the urethra into the bladder. This doesn't make a significant difference in the office setting, but when using ultrasensitive detection methods for microorganisms, one can be easily misled. The only way to eliminate this possible source of error is to perform a suprapubic urine aspiration on a patient. This involves placing a long, skinny needle directly into the bladder from a position just above the pubic bone while the bladder is full. As you can imagine, there aren't too many patients who are interested in this approach.

3. If the offending microorganism resides in the bladder wall itself, one might find nothing in the urine despite Herculean efforts. The only way to get past this problem is to analyze bladder biopsies of IC patients. Bladder biopsies can certainly be obtained but, remember, bladder biopsies generally are performed during cystoscopic procedures. Depending upon the technique of biopsy used, the specimens can be contaminated during the procedure.

Due to the problems described above, no study has yet been performed that clearly demonstrates an infectious cause to interstitial cystitis. Nevertheless, interest in this possibility persists and research continues. In the meantime, many clinicians search carefully for low numbers of bacteria that may be present in the urine of IC patients and they provide therapy based upon those findings.

Autoimmunity

To understand the process of autoimmunity, one needs a basic understanding of the immune system. Stated most simply, the immune system is designed to protect us from infection or from the introduction of abnormal cells (such as cancer cells) into our bodies. The way that our bodies accomplish this task is quite complex but essentially involves three components: specialized cells, antibodies, and other chemicals that stimulate or regulate inflammation. Together, these three parts of our immune system help rid our bodies of foreign and potentially harmful invaders.

Autoimmunity implies that "the system" has gone a bit haywire whereby the body's immune system believes that its own cells are foreign bodies. The result of this misinterpretation may lead to inflammation (that is, the patient is attacked by his or her own defense mechanisms).

Literature suggesting that interstitial cystitis is linked to this autoimmune phenomenon arose in the 1930s through the 1960s. These studies noted that IC was more commonly seen in patients who had systemic lupus erythematosus (SLE—a well-described autoimmune disease), multiple allergies, and "collagen diseases" (other diseases associated with autoimmunity). Further investigations were stimulated by the findings of M. R. Silk (1970) who found antibodies in the bloodstream directed against the bladder in nine out of twenty IC patients, but none of these antibodies were found in people without IC. Since that time, a great deal of research has been directed to the issue of autoimmunity and IC, but unfortunately, much of the data has been conflicting. For example, Anderson, Parivar, Lee,

Wallington, et al. (1989) found no statistically significant difference in bladder antibodies in IC patients than in patients without IC. Furthermore, therapies typically used in the treatment of autoimmune diseases such as steroids and immunosuppressants have not been uniformly helpful in the treatment of IC.

In summary, immunological abnormalities suggesting an autoimmune process have been described in some IC patients, but autoimmunity is unlikely to be the cause of disease in most patients.

The Role of the Mast Cell

Increased numbers of mast cells (mastocytosis) have been found in many patients suffering from interstitial cystitis. These cells are normally responsible for protecting the bladder from invading organisms and serve an important role in the inflammatory process in the bladder and other areas of the body. Note: *Inflammation is not always a harmful process. Inflammation is needed to fight infection and even diseases like cancer. Problems occur when the inflammatory process becomes out of control and for no apparent reason.*

Within the mast cells are "packets" or "granules" of substances that can cause inflammation, the most notable of which is histamine. Problems seem to arise in some IC patients when these cells begin to release their histamine abnormally in a process called degranulation. To prove this point, Kastrup, Hald, Larsen, and Nielsen (1983) demonstrated high levels of histamine in the bladder walls of many IC patients. Medications that prevent mast cells from releasing histamine and other inflammation-provoking substances are frequently useful for therapy (see chapter 5, Oral Medications).

In summary, we still don't know what causes IC. Most clinicians and investigators in this field believe that there may be multiple causes, all which give rise to similar symptoms and physical findings and which we have labeled "interstitial cystitis." For that matter, many of the abnormalities discussed in this chapter may be present in the same patient, acting in unison to create symptoms (see figure 6).

So what's the point of all of these studies if we haven't found the one cause of this disease? There are two very important answers to this question:

1. Identifying abnormalities that occur only in the IC patient may allow us to develop better tests to diagnose the condition. For example, the decreased urine level of GP51, seen in most IC patients, ultimately may be used as a commercial test.

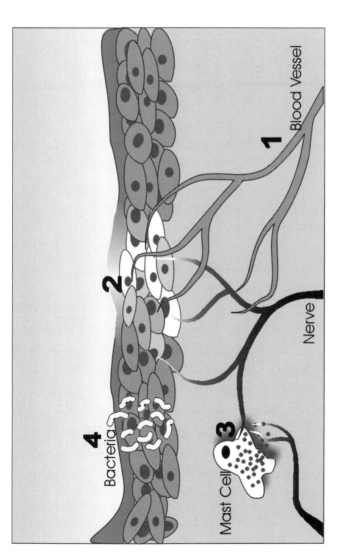

Figure 6. One or possibly many problems may account for the symptoms associated with IC. This illustration represents how multiple abnormalities might act together to cause IC. (1) represents a decrease in the blood flow to the bladder wall. This could directly affect the nerves of the bladder, leading to oversensitivity. It could also lead to abnormalities in the bladder surface cells or the production of bladder surface mucin. (2) When the nerves of the bladder are stimulated, they can secrete chemicals (like substance P) that stimulate other nerves which transmit pain. (3) These nerves also can cause inflammation. Shown here is a nerve causing a mast cell (an inflammatory cell) to release inflammation-provoking substances (like histamine). It's also possible that bacteria (4) could produce similar problems.

2. Correcting abnormalities that are found in the IC patient may lead to symptom improvement or even to cure.

These two answers emphasize just how important it is to continue research dedicated to our understanding of IC. A better understanding of the disease ultimately results in better methods of diagnosis and treatment.

Chapter 4

Medical Conditions Associated with Interstitial Cystitis

Other medical problems have long been known to co-exist with interstitial cystitis (IC). In 1949, in a review of 223 interstitial cystitis patients, Dr. J. Hand noted that allergies were more frequently seen in IC patients than in the general population. More recently, a 1997 study by Alagiri, Chottiner, Ratner, Slade, et al. described other illnesses more commonly seen in IC patients. Using the National Database of the Interstitial Cystitis Association, 2,682 IC patients were reviewed (96.5 percent female, 3.5 percent male). Some of their findings can be seen in the table below:

Table 4.1: Conditions That May Coexist with IC

Disease	% of IC Patients Diagnosed with Disorder	% of Patients in the General Population with Disorder
Allergies	40.6	22.5
Irritable Bowel Syndrome	25.4	2.9
Skin Sensitivity	22.6	10.6

Vulvodynia	10.9	15*
Fibromyalgia	12.8	3.2
Migraine Headaches	18.8	18
Asthma	9.2	6.1

* This likely represents an overestimation of this condition in the general population. Furthermore, although 10.9 percent of IC patients in this study were diagnosed with vulvodynia, 25 percent had symptoms suggestive of this problem.

Although the prevalence of inflammatory bowel diseases (such as Crohn's disease or ulcerative colitis) and systemic lupus erythematosus (SLE—an autoimmune disease characterized by problems in many organ systems) was low, they were still 100 and 30-50 times the prevalence rates seen in the general population, respectively.

In most instances, problems like allergies, migraines, asthma, and sensitive skin tended to exist prior to the symptoms of IC. Conversely, fibromyalgia and chronic fatigue syndrome tended to occur after the onset of interstitial cystitis.

Some of the problems noted above, particularly fibromyalgia and vulvodynia, can be terribly incapacitating. The symptoms of these diseases sometimes predominate over those of the bladder problem. As you can imagine, these other diseases can also play a role in worsening the symptoms of interstitial cystitis. Treatment of these disorders is therefore just as important as treatment for IC. We will now take a closer look at some of these problems and at the rudiments of their medical care.

Vulvodynia

The term *vulvodynia* means pain in the vulva, the entire female external genital region (see figure 3). The pain that is sensed is usually described as "soreness, burning, twisting, or throbbing" as opposed to vaginal itching. The evaluation, treatment, and overall medical interest in vulvodynia have taken a path remarkably similar to that of interstitial cystitis. Vulvar pain has been described since the late 1800s and early 1900s, but, as with many female-related medical issues of unclear origin, it was put on the back burner until renewed interest developed in the 1970s. That renewed interest blossomed into a workshop sponsored by the National Institutes of Health held in 1997 where current knowledge on the subject was reviewed and plans for future research in the field were discussed.

Multiple ways to subclassify vulvodynia have been proposed. The subclassification system listed below is relatively straightforward. It divides the problem into two distinct categories:

1. *Vulvodynia related to infections or skin diseases.* Vulvar diseases in this group include herpes infections, severe fungal infections, thinning and/or cracking of the vaginal surface due to estrogen loss (after menopause or removal of the ovaries), skin diseases like lichen sclerosis or lichen planus. C. M. Ridley, in an excellent review of the subject (1998), describes a disease called *cyclical vulvitis* in this category. Cyclical vulvitis, as the name implies, refers to the patient who has symptoms that come and go. These patients often respond to long-term anti–*Candida* therapy. (*Candida* is the most common yeast form seen in vaginal yeast infections.) When symptoms persist despite what appears to be adequate therapy for the specific problem, patients are often reclassified into the category below, *dysesthetic vulvodynia.*

2. *Vulvodynia unrelated to any obvious infection or skin disease.* This group can be broken down further into two groups. When IC patients have vaginal pain of unclear origin, they most frequently fall into either of these categories.

   * *Dysesthetic Vulvodynia* (originally described as "*Essential Vulvodynia*"). This problem is characterized by constant vulvar pain (usually burning) and is most commonly seen in postmenopausal women. The pain is usually not worsened by sexual intercourse and examination rarely demonstrates a specific region of tenderness. Pain sometimes extends beyond the vaginal region, radiating to the groin or inner thighs. It appears that the pain is derived from the nerves themselves. In fact, it's not unusual for patients to suffer from other chronic neurological types of problems such as glossodynia (a burning or painful tongue) or chronic facial pain.

   * *Vulvar Vestibulitis Syndrome (VVS).* Patients in this group are usually young and have faced many of the same problems faced by the IC patient—multiple doctor visits without a clear-cut strategy for evaluation or care. Interestingly, this type of vulvodynia is the most common type linked to interstitial cystitis. Unlike dysesthetic vulvodynia, the vulva hurts when it's touched. Patients often complain that their vaginal opening feels as though someone had taken sandpaper to the area and

began rubbing. Most patients complain of terrible pain with sexual intercourse in the area of vaginal penetration, called *entry dyspareunia*. It's usually uncomfortable to wear tight pants. Using tampons is just about impossible. In many instances, there's a great amount of overlap between the symptoms of dysesthetic vulvodynia and VVS, making the diagnosis less than clear-cut. The cause of VVS disease is unknown. There has been some speculation that the disease might be related to an allergic event or an autoimmune process. Recent studies by Bohm-Starke, Hilliges, Falconer, and Rylander (1998) demonstrated increased numbers of nerve fibers in the vaginal walls of VVS patients when compared to patients without VVS.

* When the clinician examines the region, redness can sometimes be seen in specific areas (sometimes called *"focal vulvitis"*). A cotton-tipped swab is usually stroked along different areas of the vulva to determine the location of pain. The regions of redness often correspond to pain sites; however, sometimes areas of tenderness are found without any redness.

Treatments Available for Vulvodynia

The vast majority of clinicians who treat interstitial cystitis are urologists; however, few urologists specialize in the management of vulvodynia. If you or your urologist feel that specific vaginal-based pain is present, further gynecological or dermatological evaluation is definitely indicated. The first step in evaluation is to rule out easily treatable diseases that can cause your symptoms. As with IC, vulvodynia is also a "diagnosis of exclusion."

It's important for your doctors to have a team approach. This is especially important because many of the therapies for vulvodynia overlap with therapy for interstitial cystitis. Like the Interstitial Cystitis Association, the National Vulvodynia Association (NVA) can be of great help to the newly diagnosed vulvodynia patient. The NVA is a nonprofit organization that began in 1994. Their goal is to educate patients and the public at large about the disease, to promote research, and to work with other health organizations to determine vulvodynia's relationship to other diseases. They are a wonderful resource for patients who need current information regarding all aspects of vulvar pain, from possible causes to treatments. They promote self-help strategies to deal with both the physical and secondary emotional components of vulvodynia. The NVA also provides a support network for interested members. Contact information for the NVA will be found in chapter 11, Support for the Interstitial Cystitis Patient.

The Treatment of Vulvar Vestibulitis

As with any medical disease, treatments generally proceed from the least invasive forms of care to the most aggressive. The following list of therapies is presented in that context:

1. **Clothing.** Avoid tight fitting undergarments and pants. Most patients avoid tight-fitting clothing just because it hurts, but it's surprising to see how many people persist with this practice, thereby worsening their symptoms. Cotton underwear and pants seem to be the best.

2. **Avoid certain bathroom toiletries.** Avoid using douches, bath oils, or vaginal deodorants. Many patients with VVS have sensitivities to these types of products.

3. **The cold pack.** When symptoms act up, a cold pack can be placed in the area of the vulva. A commercially available cold pack can be used. Alternatively, ice can be put into a plastic bag or condom, wrapped in a thin cloth, and applied to the area. The cold pack can be applied to the vulva for fifteen minutes, then taken off for fifteen minutes. The process is repeated until the acute pain settles down. The important point here is to keep the vulva cold but dry.

4. **Vulvar anesthetics.** 2 percent to 5 percent lidocaine jelly or other topical anesthetics can be applied on an "as needed" basis. This can sometimes make the difference between having or not having sexual intercourse. On the matter of sexual intercourse, vaginal lubrication is extremely important. K-Y Jelly is irritating to some VVS patients. Alternatives to this product include vegetable oil and Astroglide®.

5. **The effect of urine on the vulva.** It appears that some patients are particularly sensitive to just a few drops of urine in the vulvar region. Many of these people seem to benefit from a light coating of petrolatum (Vasoline) to this area.

6. **The role of urinary oxalate.** In 1991, Solomons, Melmed, and Heitler reported about a patient who suffered from

vulvar vestibulitis who had failed multiple treatments for her condition. The patient was found to have periodically high levels of oxalate in her urine. She was treated with calcium citrate, a medication used to modify the production of oxalate crystals. After three months, her symptoms subsided and after one year, she was pain-free. When the calcium citrate was stopped, her symptoms resumed and visa versa. This case report set off a flurry of interest in low oxalate diets and indeed, some patients seem to have benefited from such diets. The most recent well-conducted study to evaluate the role of calcium oxalate and vulvar pain was done by Baggish, Sze, and Johnson in 1997. They evaluated 130 consecutive patients with VVS and 23 volunteers who had no symptoms of vulvar pain. The investigators tallied the urinary oxalate concentration of these people for 24 hours and found that urinary oxalate concentrations were actually higher in the asymptomatic people than in the VVS patients. Nevertheless 59 patients who were found to have periodically high levels of urinary oxalate were placed on an "antioxalate regime" including a low oxalate diet and calcium citrate (400 mg taken three times per day). Twenty-four percent of these patients noted symptom improvement within three months; however, only 10 percent were able to have pain-free sexual intercourse.

7. **The role of estrogen loss.** Estrogen loss after menopause or ovary removal has the potential to worsen any preexisting vulvar pain. Many patients with VVS simply cannot tolerate topical estrogen creams. Many gynecologists or dermatologists who deal with VVS on a routine basis have developed their own formulations of estrogen cream that can be helpful. The Estring® is a relatively new way to administer estrogen to the vaginal lining. The device is a small flexible ring that is inserted high in the vagina and constantly releases estrogen for three months. It is then replaced. Some patients find this less irritating than estrogen cream. Others feel uncomfortable with the ring in place. Alternatively, oral estrogen replacement is sometimes administered.

8. **Oral medications for VVS.** Much of the therapy for VVS centers upon medications that decrease nerve oversensitivity. Most of these medications are identical to those used in the management of interstitial cystitis. Commonly used agents include low doses of tricyclic antidepressants such as amitriptyline or antiseizure medications like gabapentin.

These medications are not dispensed for their originally intended purposes (treatment of depression or seizures). They're given because of their ability to block the transmission of pain in the nervous system. These medications are reviewed in detail in chapter 5, Oral Medications.

9. **Local injections with alpha interferon.** Vulvar vestibulitis syndrome (VVS) was originally though to occur due to a subclinical viral vaginal infection (the infectious organism was thought to be the human papilloma virus, an organism that is commonly sexually transmitted). Vaginal injections with alpha interferon (an agent that activates the immune system) are sometimes used to treat these infections and that's exactly what was done to these patients. Beneficial results were seen in some patients, and alpha interferon therapy then became popular for treating VVS. The injections are typically administered into the painful area(s) three times per week for four weeks. Patients often experience flu-like symptoms along with the therapy. The onset of symptom improvement can take days to months. Therapy is judged to be a failure if no improvement occurs by three months. Most patients report short-lived improvement in symptoms. Twenty percent of patients demonstrate long-term symptom improvement.

10. **The role of steroids.** Steroids have been used either as a topical preparation applied to the vulva or as injections to the affected regions. This type of therapy is usually used for short periods of time. That's because steroids, although helpful at reducing inflammation, also can thin the lining of the vulva.

11. **Dealing with the pelvic floor.** Spasm of the muscles lining the floor of the pelvis is a common problem seen in the vulvodynia patient. In fact, sometimes the largest component of vaginal pain that the patient perceives is derived from this muscle group. The term "vaginismus" has been used in the past to describe this condition; however, we usually use the broader term, pelvic floor dysfunction, today (this topic is described in greater detail in the next section). Glazer, Rodke, Swencionis, Hertz, et al. (1995) and Glazer (1998) have demonstrated that therapy such as biofeedback, when applied to the pelvic floor muscles, can result in symptom improvement.

12. **Surgery.** Procedures to remove the "sensitive" tissue have been helpful in some patients who have not responded to

more conservative methods. Procedures range from *vestibu-loplasty* (excision of a very small region of the vestibule; see figure 3) to a procedure called *total vestibulectomy* (removal of the entire vestibule). When the later surgery is performed, the lining of the vagina that normally sits behind the vulva is advanced forward. The success rate of these procedures has been reported to be about 85 percent. That sounds like a pretty high number, but you should know that there are potential problems:

* Procedures like total vestibulectomy are not commonly performed in routine gynecological practice. The 85 percent success rate discussed above was generated by gynecological surgeons who have performed these surgeries many times. If you're thinking about undergoing such a procedure, make certain that your surgeon has had a good amount of previous experience.

* The symptoms of VVS and dysesthetic vulvodynia (constant vulvar burning) can overlap, so the diagnosis isn't always clear-cut. The problem here is that vestibulectomy is not usually a procedure that will help the patient who has dysesthetic vulvodynia. Therefore, patients who have characteristics of both forms of vulvodynia are less likely to experience a good result from surgery.

* Long-term follow-up from these surgical procedures is unknown. It's always possible that the pain could return months or years later.

Treatment of Dysesthetic Vulvodynia

The treatments for dysesthetic vulvodynia and VVS are identical except that patients who have dysesthetic vulvodynia don't seem to respond very well to either surgery or to injection with alpha interferon.

Pelvic Floor Dysfunction

Interstitial cystitis is rarely *only* a bladder problem. Problems in other organ systems are common. One striking example of such an occurrence is abnormal activity of the pelvic floor muscles, broadly termed pelvic floor dysfunction (PFD). Pelvic floor dysfunction is seen in about 70 percent of IC patients and can worsen symptoms. Often some of the most pronounced symptoms of IC derive from abnormal muscle activity in this region, rather than from the bladder. Pelvic floor dysfunction has been given many names over the past 100 years such as proctalgia fugax, levator ani syndrome, prostatodynia, and vaginismus.

What Are the Pelvic Floor Muscles?

The pelvic floor comprises a large and complex group of muscles and fascia (dense tissue that covers these muscles) which acts as a type of hammock on the floor of the pelvis). The term "complex" for these muscles is probably an understatement. Most important is their role in supporting the pelvic organs in their normal positions. Problems with this role as the "suspenders" of the pelvis can lead to any of the following disorders:

Urinary Incontinence

Urinary incontinence can be defined as the unwanted leakage of urine. It can be caused by a variety of problems but one of the most common types is related to poor support from the pelvic floor muscles and is called "stress urinary incontinence." The term "stress" relates to actions that put more pressure on the bladder, like coughing or sneezing, sometimes even laughing. It has nothing to do with your life's stresses. (Of course, I think that most people would agree that this problem can be a bit stressful itself.) Your ability to hold urine in your bladder without leakage at these times is very dependent upon the position of the bladder and urethra in your pelvis. When the muscles are weakened, this positioning can change and allow leakage to occur.

Cystocoele

Weakness of the pelvic floor can allow the bladder to "drop" into the vagina. When performing a pelvic examination, the examiner can see a bulge in the wall of the vagina which represents the bladder pushing into this region (see figure 5). Usually this is more prominent with straining. Most people who have cystocoeles have no symptoms. In some instances, cystocoeles can cause discomfort and may be associated with stress urinary incontinence. A cystocoele can also prevent the adequate emptying of the bladder because urine often remains in the sac that is created. When this occurs, bacteria that occasionally gain entrance into the bladder (and are normally voided out) can multiply and start a bladder infection. When very large, a cystocoele can actually block the flow of urine by kinking the urethra, much like kinking a garden hose will stop the flow of water.

Rectocoele

This is almost the identical problem as the cystocoele; however, in this case, the *rectum* is bulging into the vagina. As with cystocoeles, patients usually don't have symptoms. When large, rectocoeles can be associated with constipation. This occurs because the stool may collect in the vaginal bulge rather than passing through the anus (see figure 5).

Vaginal Vault Prolapse

As the name indicates, vaginal vault prolapse is the protrusion of the vaginal lining outside the vaginal opening. Essentially, the vagina is turned inside out. This condition has much the same symptoms and general appearance to the patient as a large cystocoele.

Rectal Prolapse

Rectal prolapse is a relatively uncommon condition where the rectum protrudes through the anus. This can be a very uncomfortable condition since the rectal lining often becomes cracked and inflamed.

Functions of the Pelvic Floor Muscles

The muscles of the pelvic floor also have important and complex "functional" roles in both continence (stool and urine) and sexual activity. In terms of the urinary tract, these muscles are part of the "external sphincter," muscles that normally maintain enough tension to block the passage of urine through the urethra. During the process of urination, they must relax while the bladder contracts in order to produce a normal urine flow.

Similar pelvic floor relaxation occurs with defecation. The complexity of the process becomes apparent if you think about your ability to relax your pelvic floor muscles in order to urinate while contracting your muscles in a different region of your pelvic floor to avoid simultaneous defecation.

For men and women the activities of the pelvic floor muscles vary during sexual intercourse in terms of relaxation and contraction, all the while having to keep enough muscle tone to prevent "accidents" during these intimate movements.

With such an intricate process, something is bound to go wrong from time to time. Dysfunction of the pelvic floor muscles takes place when the movements of relaxing and tightening become uncoordinated. For example, the muscles might not relax completely during urination. Problems that can occur when the pelvic floor muscles don't function properly include the following:

Pelvic Pain

Spasticity of the pelvic floor muscles, just as with any other muscle of the body may be associated with pain. The discomfort is often described as pressure, tightening, pinching, pulling, sometimes even as burning. The problem may be associated with lower back pain since some of the muscles of the pelvis extend into that region.

Poor Urinary Stream

Patients with pelvic floor dysfunction have their bladder and the muscles of the pelvic floor "fighting" with one another. The bladder is trying to push urine out while the pelvic floor muscles are trying to keep the urine in. The result is often a poor urine stream. Many patients describe a time lag between attempting to urinate and the start of the urine flow. Many patients also find that their urine stream actually stops and starts along the way. Sometimes they are not certain that they've completely emptied their bladders.

Inability to Empty the Bladder

When the pelvic floor muscles contract while you urinate, two processes occur. The first is the obstruction of urine flow from the bladder. This problem alone can cause incomplete bladder emptying. However, to make matters worse, contraction of the pelvic floor muscles also may abort a bladder contraction, thus worsening the problem of incomplete bladder emptying even further.

Constipation and Irritable Bowel Syndrome

Just as the pelvic floor muscles may prevent the normal passage of urine, the identical process can occur with the passage of stool. Constipation is a very common problem in patients with PFD. Irritable bowel syndrome (IBS) also seems to appear frequently in these patients. Irritable bowel syndrome is a functional disorder of the intestines that can cause abdominal discomfort. It's usually characterized by alternating episodes of diarrhea and constipation.

Pain with Sexual Intercourse

As stated above, the behavior of the pelvic floor muscles during sexual intercourse involves an intricate process of relaxation and contraction. When performing a pelvic examination to determine whether pelvic floor dysfunction exists, these muscles are usually tender to mild pressure. In sexual intercourse, the penis "pushes," that is, applies pressure directly into this muscle group of the female patient. You can, therefore, well imagine how the thrusting action might cause pain or make pain worse. Patients often complain that intercourse is not painful but that their overall symptoms of pelvic discomfort worsen in a few hours to 24 hours later ("the day after" syndrome). This will be discussed further in chapter 9, Sex and Interstitial Cystitis. In the male patient, the pelvic floor muscles must vigorously contract during orgasm. In the case of PFD, pain during orgasm may be experienced.

Urinary Frequency and Urgency

Spasticity of the pelvic floor muscles frequently results in the urgent need to void but is rarely associated with urine leakage. Sometimes just treating the pelvic floor dysfunction can alleviate most if not all symptoms of urinary urgency and frequency.

Why Pelvic Floor Dysfunction Occurs

In many cases, the cause of pelvic floor dysfunction is unclear. In some instances, this type of voiding problem begins in childhood. Adults with PFD often complain of constipation and/or urinary frequency as children. For unknown reasons, the symptoms "blow up" in adulthood.

Some patients with PFD note that the problem was preceded by a urinary tract infection. The infection was treated. The burning with urination dissipated but the pelvic discomfort and need to frequently urinate continued. All the pushing and straining associated with the infection remained even after the infection was treated adequately and probably resulted in continued symptoms.

Spasticity of the pelvic floor muscles can occur in the face of any form of pelvic inflammation, whether it's associated with interstitial cystitis, vulvar pain syndromes, or gastroenterological problems.

The Vicious Cycle of Pelvic Floor Dysfunction

When you void very often and may not even feel that your bladder has completely emptied, the logical thing to do is to try and *push* that urine out. It seems logical because pushing every last drop out seems as if it will decrease the number of trips you have to make to the bathroom. Maybe it will make you feel as though your bladder finally has emptied completely. Unfortunately, this rarely occurs and may even worsen the problem. Straining seems to take those spastic pelvic floor muscles and strain them even more. This, in turn, worsens symptoms, which makes you feel like straining further. This whole process slowly escalates symptoms (see figure 7).

Managing Pelvic Floor Dysfunction

The key to managing PFD is twofold: first, the problem that incites the pelvic muscle dysfunction must be dealt with and then the pelvic floor muscles must be relaxed.

Step 1: Get Rid of Any Causative Factors

Infections. As mentioned earlier, urinary tract infections are a fairly common precipitating factor. Many patients with PFD are plagued with recurrent infections, every few weeks to a few months. The cause of these infections must be evaluated by the clinician. If the infections are uncomplicated (not associated other medical problems or unusual organisms) the clinician may start you on a course

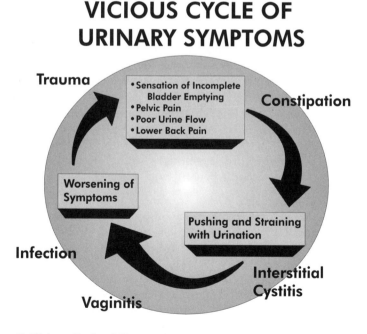

Figure 7. Vicious Cycle of Urinary Symptoms.

of *prophylactic antibiotics*. This means that an antibiotic is taken at a reduced dosage, usually at night, to *prevent* infections from occurring. If the infections are related to sexual intercourse (usually occurring 24–48 hours after intercourse), one antibiotic tablet may be taken after sex. This regime is termed *post-coital antibiotic therapy*.

Another way to manage recurrent urinary tract infections is to take the antibiotic as soon as the first symptoms appear. Many patients are placed on "self-therapy" where they are given a supply of antibiotics and are responsible for obtaining their own urinalyses and cultures. The clinician chooses the method and which antibiotic to use for recurrent infections. Many factors must be taken into consideration here, such as the patient's age, the type of bacteria found, and the patient's medical status. Other means to prevent recurrent urinary tract infections such as ingesting daily cranberry juice, blueberry juice, acidophillus, and vitamins may be somewhat helpful in preventing infections; however, acidic beverages and supplements like these can sometimes stir up the symptoms of interstitial cystitis—so be careful. Monitor your symptoms one to twelve hours after trying some cranberry juice and keep an eye out for a worsening of IC symptoms. If you're not certain of any adverse influences try again on another day.

Stress. Emotional stress is another significant problem that influences the symptoms of pelvic floor dysfunction. Just as a tension headache can be caused by tightening the muscles of the jaw and on all sides of the head, and is often prompted by stress, the identical situation appears to take place with the muscles of the pelvic floor. Many people, during stressful times, unconsciously contract their pelvic floor muscles, thereby worsening their symptoms of pelvic discomfort. Studies also suggest that the emotional impact of sexual abuse may lead to muscle-related pelvic pain and pain with sexual intercourse (Golding, Wilsnack, and Learman 1998). Stress management is clearly indicated for many patients with PFD (see chapter 10, Conservative Therapies for Interstitial Cystitis). Patients with a history of sexual abuse might benefit from counseling services.

Medical problems. Other common medical problems that appear to incite or perpetuate the symptoms of PFD include prostatitis or vaginitis. Less common problems that can initiate symptoms are radiation therapy to the pelvis, cancers of the pelvic organs, and pelvic inflammatory disease (PID) (usually related to sexually transmitted diseases). Sometimes, pelvic surgery or even minor vaginal surgery (such as a vaginal wall biopsy) can start off a cycle of symptoms. In a patient with known PFD, precautions should be taken prior to such procedures to lessen or avoid a flare-up of the condition. Interstitial cystitis or vulvar pain syndromes (generically termed vulvodynia) clearly need treatment along with accompanying PFD.

Sexual intercourse. Certain activities such as sexual intercourse may cause an exacerbation of symptoms. In women, this is probably due to intense muscle contractions in already strained and spastic muscles. Furthermore, in the patient who has some degree of discomfort with sexual intercourse, the natural tendency during penetration is to reflexively tighten her pelvic floor. When the penis enters the vaginal vault, it is met with rigid muscles—and it hurts. This causes more pain and makes her want to tighten up further the next time—if there is a next time.

The male patient with this problem has a particularly difficult time managing it since much of the muscle contraction that occurs during the orgasm is very vigorous and not under voluntary control. We'll get into the management of this problem below but it's extremely important for the male patient's partner to understand that the frequency of sexual intercourse may need to be decreased for a while until his symptoms settle down.

Exercise. Exercise is recommended, but be careful. Some exercises that seem to have nothing at all to do with the pelvic floor muscles actually do affect them. An example of this effect can be seen in the person who performs sit-ups or bench presses. The pelvic floor muscles normally tighten during these exercises because there is some abdominal straining involved. In some instances, this straining can worsen symptoms.

Step 2: Relaxing the Pelvic Floor Muscles

Learn where your pelvic floor muscles are located. In order to relax the muscles of the pelvic floor, the first order of business is to know their location. Probably the best way to accomplish this is to begin urinating, then try to stop the flow of urine. You'll notice that you have to contract a certain group of muscles to accomplish this—these are the muscles with which we're concerned. Don't repeatedly start and stop your urine stream. This can worsen your symptoms. Only do it once or twice until you feel comfortable about the location of your pelvic floor muscles. Then, don't repeat this maneuver again unless absolutely necessary. Keep track of your muscles throughout the day. Many patients note that they involuntarily contract their muscles while just sitting in a chair. If you feel that this is happening, try to consciously relax the muscles. Sometimes techniques such as biofeedback, meditation, or yoga can be of help.

Don't push with urination. Most patients with PFD try to push urine out and most interestingly, most are unaware that they're doing it. The clinician may perform a test called a "uroflow" exam that can demonstrate how much pushing is occurring. Straining with urination usually compounds the problem by causing more muscle spasms and, consequently, more symptoms—the vicious cycle again.

Avoid constipation. Constipation is a common problem in patients with PFD and probably perpetuates symptoms due to associated straining. Through extremely complex mechanisms, the nerves of the bladder and pelvic floor seem to be adversely affected when the bowel is chronically distended (which is the case with constipation). A change in the diet to include more fiber is helpful. Stool softeners such as Colace® or Metamucil® can also be used. Unfortunately, these products are often not "strong" enough to deal with the problem and laxatives are needed. We usually recommend fiber-based laxatives such as Senokot®. Constipation can also be a sign of bowel disease and, if chronic, it should be addressed by your primary care doctor or a gastroenterologist.

Take lots of warm baths. Just as one would apply a warm compress to a sore shoulder muscle, the same strategy is helpful for the muscles of the pelvic floor. When the discomfort seems to be confined to the vaginal region or the perineum (the area between the vagina or scrotum and anus) one can use a sitz bath. A *sitz bath* is a small basin that one fills with warm water that can be placed over the toilet bowl. Most patients need to take a "real" bath so that their lower abdomen is immersed in warm water. The baths should be taken for approximately fifteen minutes and here's the tough part: they should to be taken twice a day, particularly when one is just starting up with therapy. Some patients complain of vaginal soreness caused by taking so many baths. This is not a common problem, but it may be minimized by placing a colloidal oatmeal such as Aveeno® into the bathwater. Beyond this, additives such as bath oils, bubbles, etc. are not recommended. Remember, to pat yourself dry after bathing to avoid excess moisture in the vaginal region. Whirlpools are fine but be sure to keep the jets away from those sensitive areas (you'd be surprised what some people do to themselves with those jets!), since direct contact with water flow can make you tighten the muscles instead of relaxing them. Some people don't have access to a bathtub. In that event, moist heating pads are recommended. Place one pad in the region of the perineum and one on the lower abdomen. Keep in mind that the heating pads are okay but they are probably not as effective as the old-fashioned bathtub method.

Muscle relaxants can be helpful. These medications are very useful in the management of PFD. There are numerous types that can be used by the clinician. The downside of the muscle relaxants is that they can make patients sleepy. This problem can certainly limit their usefulness. We've found that diazepam (Valium®) when given in low doses (2 mg three times daily) can be extremely helpful. At low doses, it facilitates muscle relaxation and doesn't usually cause much drowsiness. If it causes too much lethargy, the tablet can be cut in half or in quarters (2 mg is the lowest dose made).

Diazepam does have some addictive potential, although very minimal at these low doses. When the symptoms of PFD slowly subside, the diazepam dose can be weaned and, hopefully, discontinued. A small percentage of patients need to be placed on a chronic low dose of a muscle relaxant under the care of a physician. Keep in mind that muscle relaxants by themselves will not treat PFD adequately. The purpose of these medications is to relax the muscles just a bit—just enough for the other items (1–4 above) to improve muscle tone and function.

The role of physical therapy. Pressing into the muscles of the pelvic floor often elicits pain. Additionally, the muscles of the pelvic floor are frequently "tight." They can feel like a taut violin string during the pelvic or rectal examination. Certain techniques of physical therapy may be helpful to reduce this muscle tension. One such technique is termed "myofascial release" in which the therapist slowly massages and stretches these muscles. The process is a slow one requiring one to three sessions per week for several weeks, depending upon the therapist's technique and the patient's response. Many patients experience an initial worsening of symptoms with myofascial release, but this usually calms down after the first few sessions. It probably occurs because a patient faced with an unusual and unfamiliar therapy may unconsciously tighten the muscles initially.

Another technique that may be helpful to the patient with PFD is transvaginal or transanal (used in the male patient) E-stim (electrical stimulation) therapy. This process involves placing a probe into the vagina or the rectum. The vaginal probe is slightly larger than a tampon. The anal probe is about the diameter of the forefinger. The probe is left in place and electrical energy is discharged into the muscles and nerves of the region. Depending upon the instrument's settings, the electrical energy can be set to slowly desensitize the nerves in the area or even cause muscle contractions to occur. This might sound like some form of torture, however, e-stim can actually be soothing to many patients. These procedures may be performed by physical therapists or in the clinician's office.

What to Expect from Therapy

Patients with pelvic floor dysfunction who are the easiest to treat usually have had their symptoms for relatively short periods of time (one to four months). It's generally more difficult to treat patients whose symptoms have been present for a long time (years) since their abnormal voiding behavior has become their new "norm." Most patients see some improvement in symptoms with the strategy outlined above within four to six weeks. This period of time can be difficult for patients because there are ups and downs along the way. Once the symptoms have settled down a bit, the therapy doesn't have to be adhered to quite as strictly. Muscle relaxants can be weaned down or discontinued. Warm baths also can be taken with less frequency. Patients should understand that although the problem seems to disappear, it can return given the right set of circumstances (for example, a recurrent urinary tract infection, a flare-up of IC, increased stress at home or in the office). Should you find that this problem is recurring, early therapy usually takes care of symptoms quickly. Remember, the sooner you start the treatment, the sooner the problem will resolve. If your symptoms don't respond to therapy to any significant degree, other problems might be the causing them and further evaluation may be needed.

In summary, PFD often accompanies interstitial cystitis as well as many other diseases of the pelvis. It's important to identify and treat the inciting problem (like IC) but also to treat the pelvic floor dysfunction.

Fibromyalgia

Fibromyalgia has been described in the medical literature for almost 200 years and it continues today as a medical enigma. Like interstitial cystitis, fibromyalgia is a disease that is mainly diagnosed on the basis of its symptoms. The disorder is characterized by diffuse and constant musculoskeletal "aching," usually concentrated in the neck, shoulders, pelvis, and back. The pain typically is worse in the morning. It tends to vary in severity throughout the day and is influenced by changes in the weather, emotional stress, and other associated medical problems. Many patients have difficulty sleeping and often awaken in the morning with fatigue. There appears to be a strong relationship between fibromyalgia and chronic fatigue syndrome (CFS) with about 90 percent of CFS patients complaining of diffuse muscle tenderness.

Fibromyalgia typically affects women in their mid-thirties. Similar to interstitial cystitis, it often begins suddenly and the severity of symptoms usually plateaus early in the course of the disease.

Also like IC, there is no specific test available to aid in diagnosis. For example, muscle biopsies and electrical studies of the muscles (electromyography) show no abnormalities. Some patients have antibody abnormalities but those patients are usually found to have other connective tissue disorders like lupus or rheumatoid arthritis. Doesn't this sound like interstitial cystitis? But, in this instance, the oversensitivity isn't in the bladder. It's probably in the muscles, connective tissue, and nerves.

In 1990, the American College of Rheumatology described the clinical criteria to establish a diagnosis of fibromyalgia. The first criterion was that pain had to be "widespread," meaning that it had to be present on the right and left sides of the body *and* above and below the waist. The second criterion was the presence of pain that could be elicited from at least 11 of 18 predefined sites on the body. Before a diagnosis of fibromyalgia can be made, other diseases that can cause similar pain must be excluded, such as hypothyroidism (the thyroid gland producing too little thyroxin); autoimmune diseases like lupus or rheumatoid arthritis; sprains; and muscle diseases like polymyalgia rheumatica.

Treatment of fibromyalgia begins with the reassurance that this is generally not a progressive problem and that there are therapies available to help. The medical therapy available to the patient with fibromyalgia includes the following:

1. **Medications to deal with any sleeping difficulties.** As previously mentioned, sleeping problems are very commonly seen in the fibromyalgia patient. Just as with interstitial cystitis, amitriptyline is one of the first-line agents for treating the fibromyalgia patient. When given in the evening hours, amitriptyline facilitates sleep and also can decrease the severity of chronic pain. Unfortunately, increasing the duration of sleep often fails to relieve the constant fatigue.

2. **Deal with depression.** People who have both fibromyalgia and IC are particularly prone to suffering from "reactive" depression. Let's face it, IC alone is bad enough. Adding another chronic painful illness has a way of dragging a person down. It's especially important to discuss these issues with your caregiver and to develop a treatment plan.

3. **Medical therapy for point tenderness.** Muscle relaxants are an important part of medical management for fibromyalgia.

Medications like cyclobenzaprine (Flexeril®) often decrease muscle pain and promote sleep. The flip side to medications such as these is that they can cause daytime fatigue. For this reason, the type of medications used and their dosages may need to be changed until the best regime is found. Nonsteroidal anti-inflammatory (NSAIDs), medications like ibuprofen, usually aren't helpful in providing pain relief. Additionally, caregivers are often reluctant to dispense high-dose, long-term therapy with these medications because of potential kidney, stomach, or liver malfunction. When long-term therapy is helpful, periodic monitoring of kidney and liver function is advised.

4. **Injection therapy of trigger points.** Some patients have significant pain relief by injecting areas of severe tenderness (trigger points) with an anesthetic. Sometimes the anesthetic is mixed with a steroid in order to decrease any inflammation that might be present. Most patients have multiple sites of tenderness, but not all of those sites can be injected. To do so would require an overdose of the anesthetic. Tender points shouldn't be injected more than one time per month or more than three times per year.

5. **Alternative strategies to medications.** Biofeedback, meditation, and physical therapy are all excellent ways to deal with fibromyalgia pain. Acupuncture has been particularly helpful for some patients. Deluze, Bosia, Zirbs, Chantrain, et al. (1992) evaluated seventy fibromyalgia patients who were assigned to an electroacupuncture (a small electrical current is applied to the acupuncture needles) or a placebo (fake electroacupuncture) group. The patients who received the "real" therapy did much better than the group who received placebo. Improvements were seen in the following categories: pain threshold, amount of analgesics required, pain scores, sleep quality, morning stiffness, and physician evaluation of pain. All of these therapies can be used by themselves or in conjunction with the other outlined forms of care.

6. **Exercise.** Aerobic training seems to be beneficial for most fibromyalgia patients. Any form of aerobic activity is acceptable. Our first choice of therapy is swimming due to its nonimpact nature. Be aware that the chlorine in the pool might worsen symptoms if vulvodynia is also present. Yoga and tai chi are other excellent forms of exercise. They're particularly helpful to many patients because they involve meditation, exercise, and stretching. Walking, jogging, or

bicycling are other good but slightly higher impact exercises. One word of caution: When starting up any exercise regime, start off *slowly*. Workouts should not be too stressful. Many a patient has pushed too hard with exercise at first. They then feel lousy and just stop practicing a discipline that could have made them feel better eventually. In general, expect to see some worsening of your symptoms before you have any improvement. It's important to keep up your exercise on a three to five times a week basis. If for any reason you stop your exercise regime for even one week, you must start off slowly again. Not to do so creates a risk of sudden increases in pain.

Where should you go for a specific exercise plan? Classes in tai chi or yoga are often held at community centers, adult education programs, and YMCAs throughout the country. Low impact aerobics classes are provided in most health clubs—but be careful. In many cases, there are some pretty aerobically fit people working out even in the beginner level classes. (I think that they're really advanced participants trying to impress the rest of the class.) Before starting a class make sure that you speak to the instructor and inform him or her of your physical condition. Alternatively, physical therapists and many personal trainers can be of help in designing a program that's right for you.

Urethral Syndrome

Urethral syndrome is a vague term used to describe urethral discomfort in the absence of a clear-cut cause. The discomfort is often described as burning. It may be present only before, during, or after urination, but in just as many instances, the pain is constant. The urethral symptoms are often accompanied by urgency and frequency of urination, pelvic pain, and pain with sexual intercourse. This is beginning to sound like IC and, in fact, *most experts in the field of interstitial cystitis consider urethral syndrome to be just another form of IC, whether or not bladder complaints are present.* As such, the term "urethral syndrome" is slowly fading out of the urological literature. The reason for adding urethral syndrome to this section is twofold. First, many clinicians still use this term; so, if you have these symptoms, you will be likely to come in contact with this terminology. Second, although much of the traditional therapy for the IC patient can be applied to the patient with urethral pain, there are often differences in care that are discussed below. Historically, urethral syndrome has been divided into two main categories:

1. **Acute urethral syndrome.** This is the sudden onset of urethral burning, along with urgency and frequency of urination. In years past, clinicians performed cultures on these patients and found no evidence of infection, but they made one very important mistake. They presumed that an infection was present only when very high numbers of bacteria were present. They didn't check for low counts of bacteria. When small numbers of bacteria were seen, they were discounted as unimportant. Today, we know that even low numbers of bacteria can cause significant symptoms in some patients. In these instances antibiotics can be curative.

   Other causes of acute urethral symptoms including sexually transmitted diseases, vaginal diseases, or vaginal infections are often found to be the cause of patient complaints. Now, you may recall that the diagnosis of urethral syndrome is based on symptoms without an obvious cause. Once the cause is known (which is true for most patients who are seen in a clinical setting today), the problem can no longer be classified as urethral syndrome. For that reason, the diagnosis of acute urethral syndrome is almost never made these days.

2. **Chronic urethral syndrome.** Patients with chronic urethral syndrome have long-standing symptoms that are identical to those in patients with the acute form. As with IC, the cause of chronic urethral syndrome is unknown. Various theories have been put forth to explain the presence of these symptoms. Some of these causation theories include the following:

   * *Fastidious organisms.* These are microorganisms that do not grow using routine culture techniques; hence they might be missed. No study to date has consistently demonstrated an infectious cause to this problem. As noted by Gittes and Nakamura (1996), a short course of antibiotics is a reasonable treatment even if the urine culture shows no obvious infection. When choosing an antibiotic, most clinicians will select those that will kill these unusual organisms. In some patients, the chosen antibiotic will deal with common sexually transmitted organisms. Sometimes, clinicians will give several different "trials" of antibiotic therapy. If no improvement in symptoms occurs, most caregivers will not prescribe any future doses of antibiotics. To continue on and on with

antibiotic therapy usually has little beneficial effect and only makes the female patient more prone to yeast infections (see "Urinary Tract Infection (UTI)" below).

* *Pelvic floor spasm.* Just as with interstitial cystitis, most patients who have urethral syndrome have pelvic floor dysfunction. Treatment of accompanying pelvic floor spasm often reduces symptoms, sometimes quite dramatically.

* *Bladder overactivity.* The symptoms of some patients with urethral syndrome appear to be related, at least in part, to an abnormally active bladder.

* *Nerve malfunction.* The urethra has many sensory nerve fibers. For unknown reasons, those nerve fibers may begin sending abnormal messages to the brain, similar to a "short circuit" seen with electrical wiring. Sensations may be transmitted even though nothing is apparently wrong with the urethra. These abnormal sensations usually feel like burning but they have also been described as pinching, pressure, and twisting. Occasionally, patients complain of the constant sensation of sexual stimulation. Sometimes the nerve problem is not at the level of the urethra at all. In these situations, the symptoms come from a higher level up in the nervous system, possibly in the brain itself, the spinal cord, or the nerves that leave the spinal cord and travel to the urethra. This type of higher level nerve malfunction is likely to be present when topical therapy to the urethra such as urethral anesthetics fail.

* *Urethral stenosis.* Urethral stenosis is a narrowing of the urethra. When this problem occurs, someone might complain of poor force to the urinary stream. Because of the blockage created by the narrowing, some patients might not empty their bladders effectively, thus any bacteria that find their way into the bladder have an easier time to multiply and cause an infection. Early studies suggested that many patients with urethral syndrome had urethral stenosis. Indeed, many patients had improvement in symptoms when the urethra was widened by a procedure called *urethral dilation* (see below). Today, we know that urethral stenosis is rarely associated with urethral syndrome. In most instances, the poor force of the

urine stream noted by many patients is due to spasm of the pelvic floor muscles or of muscles in the region of the bladder neck.

How to Deal with Urethral Syndrome

Much of the therapy that is used to treat the IC patient is also used in the management of the patient suffering from urethral syndrome. Just as with the treatment of interstitial cystitis, patients who have urethral syndrome often need multiple forms of care administered simultaneously to achieve the best results. A general listing of therapies for urethral syndrome includes the following (note that many of these therapies are discussed elsewhere in this text):

1. **Conservative management:**

   * Stress reduction

   * Dietary changes

   * Alternative approaches such as biofeedback or acupuncture

   * Support services such as the Interstitial Cystitis Association

   * Treatment of other associated problems such as vulvodynia, fibromyalgia, pelvic floor dysfunction, estrogen deficiency

2. **Oral medications:** Just as with therapy for IC, most of these medications are being used for purposes other than their original FDA indications. For example, in the treatment of urethral syndrome, Elavil® is not used as an antidepressant, but rather it's being used to relax the bladder and decrease pain.

   * Antibiotic therapy as described above

   * Alpha-blockers. These medications are commonly used in men who have a poor force to their urine stream due to growth of the prostate gland. Many practitioners also have found these medications useful for improving the poor urine flow found in female patients suffering from urethral syndrome.

* Tricyclic antidepressants for pain relief, like amitriptyline (Elavil)
* Pentosan polysulfate sodium (Elmiron®)
* Hydroxyzine
* Antiseizure medications like gabapentin (Neurontin®)
* Urinary anesthetics (such as Pyridium® and Urised®). Interestingly, these medications, often used for urethral burning, are ineffective for many patients with urethral syndrome. Nevertheless, most patients are treated with these agents at some time to determine whether any beneficial effect can be achieved

3. **Topical therapies:** Topical medications, that is, medications introduced directly into the bladder, are routinely used in the treatment of IC with pretty good results (see chapter 6, Medications Introduced into the Bladder). When treating IC in this fashion, patients are asked to hold the chosen medication in their bladders for about twenty-five minutes (if possible). We have tried to use these bladder instillations for patients with urethral syndrome, but we had less than impressive results.

   We were concerned that part of the problem with this form of care was that the medication had very little time in contact with the urethral surface. After all, the medication is usually instilled directly into the bladder. The neck of the bladder is closed while holding the medication. Therefore, the medication has no way to come into contact with the urethral surface except in that short amount of time during which the patient urinates. Because of this problem, we changed our management. At present, we instill approximately 5 cc of lidocaine® (an anesthetic) jelly mixed with a steroid (to decrease inflammation) and an antibiotic (to prevent infection from the catheterization) inserting a very small catheter into the urethra. These urethral instillations are carried out two to three times per week.

   As symptom improvement occurs, the instillations are administered with less frequency and eventually discontinued. Patients who do best with this form of treatment are those who have improvement in urethral pain derived from urinary anesthetics and those who have urethral inflammation. We have been very impressed with the results of this therapy on the small numbers of patients treated in this fashion thus far. Note: *How these patients will fair in the future is not known.*

4. **Urethral dilation:** Urethral dilation involves the insertion of progressively wider metal "sounds" (blunt-tipped metal rods) into the bladder via the urethra. This procedure is usually performed in the office setting. The urethra is anesthetized using lidocaine jelly prior to insertion of the sounds. Urethral dilation is most often performed to widen the narrowed urethra—but as you may recall, the urethra of most patients with urethral syndrome is of normal width (see the subsection on *Urethral stenosis*). So, why were the symptoms of some patients improved with urethral dilations? The answer is not clear. Possible explanations include the following:

* Many of the symptoms of urethral syndrome are often derived from spasms of the pelvic floor muscles. Urethral dilation forcibly stretches those muscles, causing them to relax.

* Urethral dilation causes temporary malfunction of the nerves of the urethra (called a *neuropraxia*), leading to a decrease in nerve sensitivity.

* Stretching of the urethra might improve drainage of infected urethral glands.

Please remember that these are only *possible* explanations for symptom improvement. None have ever been proven correct or incorrect.

An excellent article by Lemack, Foster, and Zimmern (1999) evaluated the practice patterns of 194 urologists regarding the use of urethral dilation in women with urethral syndrome. About 48 percent of physicians had used the procedure six or fewer times in their practice over the previous year while 24 percent stated that they had used the procedure over thirty times within the year. Sixty-one percent of urologists trained within the past decade had never offered urethral dilation to their urethral syndrome patients. Of those urologists who had trained more than ten years ago, only 21 percent found the procedure to be very or extremely successful. None of forty-two more recently trained urologists considered urethral dilation to be useful. In summary, there are definite doctor-age and training-related biases regarding the use of urethral dilation. It looks as if most younger urologists don't use the procedure much. What's even more interesting is the discrepancy between the published high efficacy rates for urethral dilation (that range is from 30–75 percent) and the mediocre impression of efficacy seen by community urologists.

Our approach has been to evaluate the urethra with a cystoscope in order to identify any inflammatory changes or true urethral narrowing that might be present. The passage of the cystoscope itself can sometimes result in symptom improvement, achieving results identical to urethral dilation (Rutherford, Hinshaw, Essenhigh, and Neal 1988). In the rare instance that urethral narrowing or stricture is present (this is usually noted when the cystoscope cannot be easily admitted into the bladder), urethral dilation is indicated.

Urethral dilation is also contemplated for a patient who has failed other forms of local urethral care, treatment of pelvic floor dysfunction, and so forth. Does this mean that it's wrong to perform urethral dilations as the first-line care for the patient with urethral syndrome? The answer is no. As noted in the Lemack, Foster, and Zimmern study (1999), many practitioners feel quite comfortable with this approach. These caregivers have had successes with the procedure in the past, and this has motivated them to continue this practice.

Here are some of *our* observations and advice regarding urethral dilation:

* If a cystoscopy was performed with a rigid instrument (most practitioners use flexible instruments these days) and you didn't experience symptom improvement, the chances are, urethral dilation won't help.

* If cystoscopy demonstrates an inflamed urethra, urethral dilations often make symptoms worse (at least temporarily) and they don't improve symptoms on a long-term basis.

* Most patients who improve with urethral dilations have pelvic floor muscle dysfunction, a condition we believe is better treated with muscle relaxation techniques rather than a forcible stretching. Using urethral dilation, these patients commonly have good symptom improvement, at first. Unfortunately, symptoms often recur. Another dilation is usually performed, but this time the symptoms may return more rapidly. As urethral dilations are repeated, symptoms can eventually persist despite the use of dilations.

5. **More aggressive urethral manipulation—Cryotherapy:** "Cryo" means cold. In most instances, cryotherapy involves

the destruction of tissue by freezing. Various techniques of cryotherapy have become popular in the treatment of cancer. When treating cancers, a thin metal probe (with a sharp tip) is pushed into the tumor. The probe is then cooled down to very low temperatures that actually turns the tissue into an "ice ball."

Cryosurgery is also routinely used to remove skin lesions like condyloma (venereal warts). Liquid nitrogen (a very cold liquid) is usually applied to the lesion. The area of application turns white and the lesion sheds or is cast off.

The use of cryotherapy expanded into the treatment of urethral syndrome in the 1980s. In 1984, Boreham treated 350 patients with a special cryotherapy probe. Of 111 patients who were followed up, 95 percent had symptom improvement. Ten patients required second procedures. In 1989, Sand, Bowen, Ostergard, Bent, et al. compared urethral dilation to cryotherapy. They found improvement in 91 percent of patients receiving cryotherapy and only 33 percent who underwent dilation.

These may sound like pretty spectacular results, yet cryotherapy has lost much of its appeal due to attendant problems such as urinary retention, pain, bleeding, and the return of symptoms.

Urinary Tract Infection (UTI)

Most epidemiological studies indicate that anywhere from 30–50 percent of women will develop a urinary tract infection during their lifetime. Of those that develop a urinary tract infection, about 20–30 percent will develop recurrent infections, meaning that the infections occur more than two times per year (Barnett and Stephens 1997).

Most of these infections are of the uncomplicated variety: infections that aren't associated with structural abnormalities of the urinary tract, neurological diseases, or unusual organisms. They are superficial infections that are confined to the bladder and easily treated with a wide variety of antibiotics.

The problem for the IC patient is that these infections can cause a severe flare in symptoms. For most non-IC individuals, proper antibiotic therapy results in alleviation of symptoms within one to three days. On the other hand, when an IC patient develops a UTI, the infection may be quickly eradicated, but the symptoms of urinary urgency and frequency, and pelvic pain and pressure may last for weeks. To top this off, IC patients report twice the incidence of UTI as those without IC. In order to understand how we deal with urinary tract infections, you first need to learn a little about how they occur.

What Causes a UTI?

Bacteria usually cause urinary tract infections. Infections of the urinary tract are rarely caused by other organisms such as viruses, yeast, or parasites. The most common type of bacterium that causes a bladder infection is *Escherichia coli* (*E. coli*) (85 percent of cases); however, other organisms such as *Staphylococcus saprophyticus*, *Enterococcus* sp., *Klebsiella pneumoniae*, and *Proteus mirabilis*, to name just a few, are also seen. In almost all instances, a bladder infection is not caused by an organism that you picked up from a dirty toilet seat. It actually originates from the individuals themselves. Bacteria from the rectum can slowly migrate to the vagina and probably hover around the urethral meatus (the opening of the urethra). They, then, can sometimes migrate further into the urethra and on into the bladder. We all have basic defense mechanisms against such a bacterial attack. Some of these "host defenses" include the following:

* **The lining of the vagina (the vaginal mucosa).** It's generally difficult for most bacteria to stick to the walls of the vagina. This "anti-adherence" property seems to be at least partly maintained by the presence of estrogen. Estrogen maintains the thickness, the state of the blood vessels, and the overall appearance of the vagina walls. When estrogen loss occurs, either by removal of the ovaries or by menopause, the walls can change in such a manner as to make the individual more susceptible to bladder infections. That's why some clinicians prescribe estrogen supplementation, either as a pill, topically (as a cream), or an Estring® (a soft, synthetic ring that's placed into the vagina and slowly releases estrogen) for these patients.

* **Normal vaginal bacteria.** The vagina is normally colonized by lactobacilli. These are bacteria that help to maintain the normal vaginal environment. Lactobacilli also secrete hydrogen peroxide that helps kill other potentially harmful bacteria like *E. coli*. Along with estrogen, lactobacilli help to create an acidic vaginal pH that usually keeps other types of organisms such as yeast away. By holding all the "seats" in the vagina, the lactobacilli usually crowd out any other organisms that might show up, such as *E. coli* or yeast. Lactobacilli are often killed off when broad-spectrum antibiotics (antibiotics that treat many different types of bacteria) are used to treat infections elsewhere in the body. When the lactobacilli are gone, other organisms that are resistant to those antibiotics such as yeast grow in their place and voila!— yeast vaginitis. (How to prevent this problem is discussed

below.) Spermicides used for contraception also seem to increase the likelihood of a UTI because of their ability to kill off the normal vaginal bacteria.

* **Bladder surface mucin.** This is the slimy coating of the bladder wall. Bladder surface mucin is a rather complex mixture of substances that prevents bacteria from attaching to the underlying cells of the bladder. Changes in this layer are seen in many IC patients. It's presumed that these changes account for the oversensitivity of the bladder wall observed in some individuals. No studies have been performed to see whether or not these changes correlate to a given IC patient's tendency to develop bladder infections.

* **Few receptors for bacteria on the bladder wall.** Bacteria must bind to the bladder wall prior to invasion. This binding occurs to special regions called *receptors* on the surface cells of the bladder. Those individuals who have lots of available receptors are more susceptible to bladder infections.

* **Urine factors.** The urine is usually an inhospitable place for bacteria to live. Concentrated urine seems to be the best at inhibiting bacterial growth. If one were to make recommendations *just* based upon this fact, clinicians would be telling everybody to drink sparingly since the less you drink, the more concentrated your urine will be. But, on the contrary, it's more important to drink plenty of fluids to "wash out" any bacteria that gain entry into the bladder. A more dilute urine may also lessen some IC symptoms.

* **Normal bladder emptying.** In the normal individual, the bladder empties to completion. In this way, any bacteria that happen to wander into the bladder are voided right out. Sexual intercourse commonly causes a few bacteria to be pushed up into the bladder. That's why patients who develop an infection shortly after sexual intercourse (24–48 hours) are told to urinate after sex.

Tips to Prevent and Treat Urinary Tract Infections

1. **Drink plenty of fluids.** This always creates a troubling problem for the IC patient since "the more one drinks, the more one pees." This is true but, in fact, many IC patients experience a decrease in symptoms when they increase their

fluid intake. That's probably because the bladder surface is sensitive to concentrated urine. Increasing the fluid intake allows the individual to void out any bacteria that gain entry. The most commonly asked question now is, "Then just how much should I drink?" That's a difficult question to answer since adequate fluid intake is dependent on many factors such as your overall medical condition and your level of physical activity. In general, we find the best indicator of urine concentration is its color. Dilute urine (the kind that you want to shoot for) is clear to light straw-colored. Patients who are taking vitamins or medications that change the color of the urine might have problems with this method of tracking. Sometimes stopping these agents for a few days (under proper medical supervision) and observing the urine color (with increases in fluid) can be helpful. One thing's for sure—if you feel as though a bladder infection is beginning, it's always a good idea to increase your fluid intake even beyond your normal amount.

2. **Short courses of antibiotics.** Most uncomplicated bladder infections are treated adequately with just a three-day course of antibiotics. This method of treatment became popular when it was found that this form of therapy resulted in identical cure rates to the traditional seven to ten day course of antibiotic therapy. Three days of therapy is also less likely to alter the bacteria that normally inhabit the vagina. Hence, there's a lower chance of developing a vaginal yeast infection. Some clinicians might wish to treat with longer courses of antibiotics because they feel that the infection is "complicated." Complicated infections are usually more "deep-seated" in the urinary tract. They are usually associated with unusual organisms, anatomical abnormalities (such as poor bladder emptying due to a cystocoele, or a "dropped" bladder), or neurological abnormalities.

3. **Get prompt attention for your symptoms.** The best way to get rid of the symptoms of a bladder infection is to get the infection treated quickly. By starting antibiotic therapy at the very onset of symptoms (urinary urgency, frequency, burning with urination and pelvic discomfort) the bacteria are killed before they can cause severe inflammatory changes of the bladder surface (remember, the symptoms of a UTI arise from the inflammation that the bacteria cause, not the bacteria themselves). Once severe inflammation occurs, the bacteria can still be killed but it can take a long time for the

symptoms to resolve. If the infection is treated within the first few hours of symptom occurrence, the urinary discomfort may last twelve to twenty-four hours, then fade away. When there is a delay in therapy, symptoms may last much longer. This is significantly exaggerated in the IC patient, where a flare in symptoms may last several weeks. For this reason, we are proponents of "self-therapy" for the patient who develops infections on a relatively infrequent basis. Various methods of antibiotic self-therapy exist. The protocol that is used entails the patient receiving a prescription for an antibiotic, several prescriptions for urinalysis/urine culture, and a urine culture cup. Patients are instructed to purchase the antibiotic and keep one or two tablets with them at all times. If the patient feels that a bladder infection is starting up, she urinates into the sterile container and stores it in her refrigerator. She then takes her first antibiotic tablet and continues on a three-day course of antibiotic therapy. Within twenty-four to forty-eight hours, she brings her urine to a local laboratory. The results of the urinalysis and culture are faxed to the clinician's office. Self-therapy strategies may vary greatly amongst clinicians.

4. **Try not to use a diaphragm or spermicides if your infections are related to sexual intercourse.** Many people develop a bladder infection twenty-four to forty-eight hours after sexual intercourse. Epidemiological studies have indicated that the use of the diaphragm increases the risk of urinary tract infection (Foxman and Frerichs 1985). Additionally, the spermatocide nonoxynol-9, alters the normal vaginal bacteria and thus makes it easier to develop a UTI. We find that few IC patients use a diaphragm for contraception, not because of the UTI issue but because it causes too much vaginal/bladder irritation. Nevertheless, if you use a diaphragm and your urinary tract infections seem to be related to sexual intercourse, it's best to speak with your medical caregiver about changing to some other form of contraception.

5. **A note about anal intercourse.** Some IC patients have modified their lovemaking activities to anal intercourse rather than performing vaginal penetration. If, however, you perform both anal and vaginal intercourse during the same session, it's probably best to perform vaginal intercourse first. Performing anal intercourse first creates a higher probability of carrying bacteria into the vagina and then into the urethra and bladder.

6. **Be sure to urinate after sexual intercourse.** Sexual intercourse can cause the migration of bacteria into the bladder. If this occurs and you fall asleep, you're giving any bacteria that were introduced into your bladder time to multiply. This is a big problem for those individuals who are more susceptible to bladder infections. The best way to prevent this is simply to urinate immediately after sexual intercourse.

7. **Antibiotic therapy for infections related to sexual intercourse.** Sometimes bladder infections occur after sexual intercourse even though you stay away from the diaphragm and urinate immediately after sex. When this is a constant problem, your doctor might wish to start you on a course of *post-coital antibiotic therapy.* You are given a supply of an antibiotic. One antibiotic tablet is taken after sexual intercourse to prevent infection from occurring.

8. **The use of lactobacilli.** As stated above, lactobacilli are bacteria that normally inhabit the vagina and appear to prevent vaginal yeast and bladder infections by keeping away organisms associated with those problems. Many different types of lactobacilli exist. The type of lactobacilli found in live yogurt cultures has been shown to decrease the occurrence of yeast vaginitis. Unfortunately, no study to date has definitively shown that taking lactobacilli orally or even douching with these "friendly" bacteria will prevent a bladder infection. It may very well be that some strains of lactobacilli are better at preventing a bladder infection than others. The problem right now is that we simply don't know which type is best. The strains of lactobacilli found in most commercial preparations (over-the-counter *lactobacillus acidophillus*) are unlikely to be as helpful in the prevention of a urinary tract infection as the lactobacilli that are normally found in the vagina. That's why it's so important for the individual to maintain her vaginal lactobacilli as best as possible. That means using long courses of antibiotics only when necessary; staying away from spermicides if possible; and avoiding frequent douching.

9. **The use of cranberry juice.** Cranberry juice has been a longtime folk remedy for the prevention and treatment of bladder infections. In the 1988, Schmidt and Sobota substantiated cranberry juice's beneficial effect on the urinary tract. In their studies, cranberry juice was shown to inhibit the binding of bacteria to cells found on the bladder surface. In 1994, a study by Avorn, Monane, Gurwitz, Glynn, et al. reported

that daily ingestion of about ten ounces of cranberry juice cocktail by elderly women significantly reduced the chances of finding bacteria and pus cells in their urine. Although this study did not conclusively demonstrate any decrease in the development of a *symptomatic* urinary tract infection in the group who drank cranberry juice cocktail, it did suggest that cranberry juice plays a potential role in the prevention of bladder infections. It seems as though the beneficial effect from the cranberry juice has nothing to do with the added fluid intake, the vitamin C content, or the acidity of the drink. The problem with cranberry juice for the IC patient is that it may cause a flare in symptoms. It also has lots of sugar which can promote weight gain—especially if you drink it frequently. It's unclear whether the newly created and marketed dehydrated cranberry tablets have the same effect as the unprocessed product.

10. **The use of chronic antibiotic prophylaxis.** When bladder infections recur with great frequency, the bladder barely has time to get rid of its inflammation when another infection hits. This is a potential disaster for any IC patient, and in our opinion, needs to be treated aggressively with appropriate antibiotic therapy. The most common approach to dealing with rapidly recurring bladder infections is chronic antibiotic prophylaxis. This means that the patient takes an antibiotic tablet each night. The dose of antibiotic is low but high enough to keep infections from occurring. By keeping infections away for a long time, the bladder has a chance to heal and the patient doesn't have to suffer from the rapid cycling of UTI symptoms. The goal of therapy is to keep the antibiotic dose as low as possible while keeping infections away. If infections seem to occur only around the time of the menstrual flow, prophylactic antibiotics can be dispensed just at that time. Alternatively, if a patient hasn't had an infection for a while on her nightly dose of antibiotic, the clinician might wish to see if she remains infection-free on an every-other-night dosing schedule. The clinician might eventually wish to stop the antibiotic completely.

After all that's been previously said about antibiotics and how they can alter the normal vaginal bacteria, you should be wondering by now how chronic antibiotic prophylaxis affects the chance of developing vaginal yeast infections. In fact, low doses of antibiotics rarely harm the normal vaginal bacteria (lactobacilli). Many of the antibiotics administered for chronic prophylaxis such as nitrofurantoin (Macrodantin®, Macrobid®) are not secreted in vaginal fluid. The fact that these medications are not secreted in vaginal fluid means that the lactobacilli of the vagina are not affected. This minimizes the risk of subsequent yeast infections. They are excreted in the urine and therefore only affect bacteria found there.

11. **Urinary anesthetics and medications that relax the bladder.** The burning with urination that is usually associated with a urinary tract infection can often be alleviated with the use of urinary anesthetics such as phenazopyridine hydrochloride (Pyridium®). Likewise, the severe urgency and frequency of urination may not all be related to interstitial cystitis. When a bladder infection is present, the bladder sometimes contracts uncontrollably. If this is occurring, the problem can be diminished with the use of anticholinergic medications (see chapter 5, Oral Medications). Anticholinergic medications must be administered with caution to patients who don't empty their bladders completely. By relaxing the bladder further, the bladder might retain even more urine.

12. **Watch out for associated pelvic floor dysfunction.** The symptoms of a bladder infection often cause patients to bear down when urinating. This maneuver (many individual don't even know that they're doing this) ultimately can result in spasm of the pelvic floor muscles. Dysfunction of these muscles can lead to more symptoms of pelvic pain as well as to urinary urgency and frequency. One needs to be aware of this potential problem. Avoid giving into the temptation to squeeze that urine out. Frequent warm baths also can be helpful at calming any muscle spasm. This problem is discussed in detail elsewhere in this chapter.

Interstitial Cystitis and Pregnancy

Unpublished studies conducted by the Interstitial Cystitis Association suggest that the symptoms of interstitial cystitis actually decrease during the first two trimesters of pregnancy.

Urinary frequency and pain are said to increase during the third trimester, presumably due to pressure from the expanding uterus. (Of course, an increase in urinary frequency during the third trimester is common in non-IC individuals for the same reason.) Our observations have not been as favorable. We've seen the majority of patients have some degree of symptom worsening throughout their pregnancies, most likely related to the necessary discontinuance of their oral medications. Only selected medications such as narcotics can be dispensed with safety and, of course, these medications must be monitored with care. Additionally, most obstetricians and midwives do not recommend taking warm baths due to fears of raising the temperature of the pelvic contents too high for a developing fetus. In general, pregnancy can be a tough time for the IC patient; however, most patients make it through without any problems. Conservative management including yoga, meditation (relaxation techniques) and self-hypnosis, acupuncture, dietary changes, avoidance of constipation, and the possible intermittent use of narcotics is usually the best way to go.

Make sure to take a Lamaze class if you're planning to have a vaginal delivery. You might think that a cesarean section is a better way to deliver your baby than a normal vaginal delivery. After all, a C-section avoids a possible episiotomy (an incision created to increase the size of the vaginal opening, performed to avoid an uncontrolled tear in this region during the delivery) and further pressure upon your bladder and pelvic floor muscles.

In reality, no study to date has ever evaluated the benefits and downsides of each method of delivery for the IC patient. Our stance has been to advocate vaginal deliveries because we've observed that the vast majority of IC patients do just fine with this approach. Patients who would probably do better with C-section are those who have vulvodynia associated with IC. Certainly, other obstetrical or medical issues might make a C-section the procedure of choice.

If You're Going to Have a C-Section

If a C-section is performed, a Foley catheter is placed into the bladder at the time of the procedure. A "Foley" is a narrow tube that is inserted into the urethra and then into the bladder. The catheter remains in the bladder due to a small balloon that is inflated at its tip. The Foley catheter is connected to a drainage bag that collects urine. Initially, the catheter is placed so as to empty the bladder and to keep it empty during the surgical procedure. The patient's urine output can be carefully watched after the delivery. Overall, the Foley makes the C-section safer for the patient. Because the catheter remains in the bladder for only a short period of time, a resultant urinary tract infection is unlikely (long-term catheterization is almost always associated with bacteria in the urine). The catheter is removed by deflating the balloon through a small side port on the catheter. You might have some burning associated with urination the first few times after the catheter is removed. That usually settles down over the course of a day.

If You're Going to Have a Vaginal Delivery

Most pregnant IC patients undergo vaginal deliveries. As mentioned above, most patients do nicely with this approach but many patients have concerns about possibly needing a catheter; or how an episiotomy might affect their symptoms. Note that most patients will not need the insertion of a catheter into the bladder. When a catheter is inserted, it's usually because the patient can't urinate. *Urinary retention* (the inability to empty the bladder well) can happen for a variety of reasons, but most commonly it occurs due to poor bladder function after delivery. Bladder function can be impaired from pain medications or anesthesia. Another problem that can impair bladder emptying after delivery is pelvic floor spasticity, where the urine is held back by inappropriate tightening of the muscles that ordinarily maintain your urinary continence (see "Pelvic Floor Dysfunction" earlier in this chapter).

Many patients experience discomfort in the vagina, the perineum (the area between the vagina and anus), and the region around the anus after delivery. Some patients even develop hemorrhoids at this time. All of this prompts more pelvic floor spasticity often to the point where the muscles of the pelvis tighten and do not allow urine to void efficiently. If you just can't urinate and you're developing more pelvic pain due to distention of your bladder, you need a urinary catheter. You might want to ask your medical caregiver if an anesthetic jelly is available. This jelly is not found routinely on obstetrical floors so it might require some preplanning. The anesthetic jelly is inserted into the urethra prior to catheter placement and often makes the catheterization more tolerable. The urine is drained and the amount of urine obtained is recorded. The amount of urine that is drained from the bladder is used to determine how long the catheter must be left in place. If only moderate amounts of urine are drained (which is usually the case), the catheter is left in place for a day or two. Patients are then given a "voiding trial," to prove that they can urinate without difficulty.

Many, if not most, patients undergoing a vaginal delivery receive an episiotomy. An episiotomy is performed by creating an incision from the back portion of the vaginal opening into the perineum (the region between the vagina and anus). Like any minor surgical procedure, the episiotomy is associated with some postoperative pain. That pain, in addition to the trauma of childbirth, can stir up pelvic floor spasm and the overall symptoms of IC. Keep in mind that this can be partially offset by the fact that the bladder pressure may significantly dissipate after the birth of the baby.

Chapter 5

Oral Medications

Oral medications when used alone or in combination with other medications will improve symptoms in most interstitial cystitis (IC) patients. That's not to say that patients will have no symptoms at all—but they may be improved to a point where they wish to hold off on further, more invasive, therapy. Most of the medications used cause few significant side effects. When significant side effects do occur, it's important to know how to minimize them or avoid them altogether. Often, knowing these "tricks" can make the difference between discontinuing or taking a potentially very helpful drug.

Before proceeding with a listing of medications, please note that most of the medications listed here have been used in medical practice for many years but for different purposes. They were FDA (Food and Drug Administration) approved for those other medical problems but *not* for IC. In the meantime, much literature has been amassed within the past fifteen years, detailing the benefits of these medications for IC sufferers and they should be well-known to clinicians treating IC patients.

This chapter is written only as a guide to the medications. The selection, dosages, and duration of therapy are up to the individual clinician. Many factors go into the final medical treatment plan. Some of these factors include the following:

* The clinician's experience with the medication

* Results and side effects on other patients treated with the medication

* The specific symptoms of the patient

* The clinician's interpretation of literature regarding the medication

* Allergies and sensitivities that the patient has had in the past

* Other medical problems the patient might have

* Other medications the patient is taking

* The patient's experiences with a specific medication in the past. For example, if the patient has taken a medication in the past and has had no benefit, the clinician might wish to avoid that medication again. This can get complicated when dealing with the IC patient because, occasionally, medications that have no effect at one point in time seem to work very well at other times

* The cost of the medication

With all these factors to consider, the decision regarding which medication(s) to choose can be complex. Quite frankly the decision is not always correct the first time around. Medications and dosages may need to be changed due to side effects or poor responses. It can be very frustrating for patients since they have to live with their symptoms while these issues are being sorted out. Try not to become discouraged. Fortunately, most patients ultimately find the medical therapy that helps. Patients and their clinicians should decide if and when other interventions are needed (such as medications that can be introduced into the bladder). As a final note, it is certainly possible that your medical practitioner may recommend a medication that is not covered here. This list is not meant to be exhaustive. Rather, it reviews the most commonly used oral agents in the management of IC.

Medications Thought to Coat the Bladder Surface

The bladder surface is normally protected by a thin but important lining called bladder surface mucin. Abnormalities of this lining have been demonstrated in IC and are thought to result in heightened sensitivity of the bladder wall in some patients (see chapter 3, What Causes Interstitial Cystitis?). Medications that improve the quality of bladder surface mucin therefore have the potential to improve the symptoms of IC patients.

Pentosan Polysulfate Sodium (Elmiron®)

Elmiron is a relatively new addition to the treatment of interstitial cystitis and is the only oral medication to date that has FDA approval specifically for the treatment of IC symptoms. Elmiron is a mild anticoagulant (blood thinner) when administered intravenously but when taken orally it has little of this effect. Elmiron is considered to be a *heparinoid*. That means that it's very similar in molecular structure to heparin sulfate, a normal component of bladder surface mucin (the protective coating that lines the bladder surface). When taken orally, a small percentage of the medication is excreted into the urine unchanged. Although it has not yet been experimentally proven, it's thought that the medication binds to the bladder surface and enhances its protective lining. The FDA-approved dosage for Elmiron is 100 mg, taken three times daily.

Elmiron appears to improve symptoms in 35–40 percent of patients. Studies are currently ongoing to determine whether higher doses will result in even further symptom improvement. The biggest therapeutic problem with Elmiron is that it can take three to six months to have its desired effect. That can be a big problem for patients because it means that they might have to live with their symptoms for a long time before the drug's ultimate effect is known. It has therefore become rather common for clinicians to begin patients on Elmiron along with other medical therapy. If another medication is to be used, we usually space the initiation of therapies by about two weeks. In this manner, should side effects occur, the time differential allows identification of the troublesome medication.

Problems with the medication may include:

1. **Stomach upset.** This is probably the most common complaint of patients regarding Elmiron. A recent finding has been that the capsule itself may be the culprit. For these patients, it's advised to mix the capsule's contents into a glass of water and drink it down.

2. **Hair loss.** This problem is not common. It occurs in about 3–4 percent of patients. When it does occur, it usually causes patches of hair loss. Unfortunately, at the very mention of this issue many patients become leery about starting therapy. Additionally, as soon as patients begin taking the medication, most immediately start to look at their hairbrushes. What do they see? They see their normal hair loss that has nothing to do with the medication, but they interpret this as a side effect and stop taking potentially helpful treatment. A

good suggestion here would be to hold off taking your medication for about one to two weeks. During that time, brush your hair each day and monitor how much hair is "normally" lost each day. Then you would have a baseline. If you do that, when you are taking Elmiron, you can judge more accurately whether the medication is causing significant hair loss.

3. **Increased bruisability.** Elmiron is a very weak "blood thinner" when taken orally. A small percentage of patients may develop this problem. In these instances, the medication usually needs to be discontinued.

4. **Liver function abnormalities.** Another rare problem with Elmiron is a change in liver function. This potential effect can be monitored with occasional blood tests.

5. **Cost.** Elmiron is a relatively recent addition to the medications available in the management of IC. Currently there is no generic form of this medication available. The price varies from region to region but is in the range of about $160–200 per month.

Chondroitin Sulfate/Glucosamine

These are agents that can be obtained in health food stores. Chondroitin sulfate is actually one of the large molecules that comprise bladder surface mucin, the coating of the bladder wall that appears to protect the underlying bladder wall. Most literature related to these large carbohydrates relates to the treatment of arthritis. There have been no clinical studies undertaken to determine the correct dosage or efficacy of these medications in the management of IC, only anecdotal reports. They are similar in molecular structure to heparin sulfate and Elmiron but that doesn't in any way mean that they function in a similar fashion.

Antidepressants

Various types of antidepressants have become cornerstones in pain management centers around the world, not because they make you "happier" but because they actually reduce pain.

Amitriptyline (Elavil®)

Amitriptyline's initial use was in the treatment of depression. Chemically, it belongs to a group of medications called *tricyclic antidepressants.* These drugs, when administered in relatively low doses, serve an important role in the management of IC. They are also used extensively in pain management centers for the treatment of pain related to other diseases. Although other medications in this group can improve the symptoms of IC, amitriptyline has been studied in the greatest detail.

The obvious questions that now arise are these: Why are you giving me an antidepressant to treat my symptoms? Do you think that my problem is all in my head? In a word, the answer is: No. The medication is not being given for a psychological disturbance. Amitriptyline and other medications of this sort have other effects that can improve the symptoms of IC apart from their impact on depression. Furthermore, the doses that are administered are usually lower than the doses given for major depressive illness. Generic forms of amitriptyline are available. The medication is therefore not terribly expensive.

Amitriptyline's positive impact appears to stem from the following factors:

1. **It causes some sleepiness.** For the average patient taking the medication during the day, this is not such a great quality. However, that's not usually how these medications are administered to IC patients. We use this "side effect" to help patients sleep better. Taking a tablet at about 7:00 P.M. often helps a great deal. It's not uncommon to see a patient who "normally" awakens eight times per night and reduce that frequency to three or four times.

2. **These medications block the transmission of pain.** This phenomenon appears to occur in the spinal cord and brain. The exact mechanism is not completely understood but this quality makes these medications useful for other pain syndromes, too.

3. **Bladder relaxation is promoted.** About 10 percent of IC patients have some degree of bladder overactivity. This means that the bladder contracts when the patient doesn't want to urinate. This can result in urgency and frequency of urination and sometimes even urine leakage. Many of these medications have anticholinergic (bladder relaxing) qualities that can improve this problem.

4. **Antihistamine effect.** This is an effect that's similar to hydroxyzine (see below). Amitriptyline, in this instance, can decrease inflammation.

The dose that's administered usually ranges from 10–75 mg at night. The dose usually starts at 10–25 mg and is gradually increased until the patient starts to feel better. Symptom improvement takes about one to three weeks to occur. Amitriptyline seems to work better in patients who have bladder capacities greater than 600 cc under anesthesia (most IC patients have slightly higher bladder capacities) (Hanno and Wein 1991).

Side Effects

Amitriptyline can have side effects that preclude its use in some patients. Here's a list of potential problems associated with amitriptyline and how they often can be solved.

1. **Morning lethargy.** Amitriptyline may be very helpful at letting patients sleep better at night but sometimes this effect lasts into the morning hours. This can be particularly disconcerting to the patient who needs to wake up early and has an active morning ahead either at work, with the kids, or driving. Many patients describe this as a "hangover" effect. It's frequently due to taking the medication too late at night. The problem is often improved considerably by taking the tablet at dinnertime (7:00 P.M.) and not after the late, late, late show.

2. **Constipation.** One of amitriptyline's useful qualities is its ability to slow down bladder activity. Unfortunately, this ability also may slow down the activity of your intestines, thus causing constipation. This is potentially a big problem because constipation and associated straining may worsen pelvic floor problems (see chapter 4 for a discussion of pelvic floor dysfunction). For that matter, distention of the rectum with hard stool can cause pelvic pain. It's therefore wise to treat the constipation prior to starting a course of amitriptyline.

3. **Dry mouth.** Just as amitriptyline can slow down bowel function, it also slows down the output of saliva from our salivary glands. This problem varies from patient to patient but is usually not very severe when it occurs. Switching to another tricyclic antidepressant can frequently alleviate this side effect.

4. **Urinary retention.** The ability of amitriptyline to relax the bladder can be helpful to many patients but sometimes the medication's a bit too efficient. Occasionally, patients taking amitriptyline will notice that their urine stream slows down.

Rarely, a patient will have such sensitivity to amitriptyline that he or she can't urinate at all, and needs to be catheterized until bladder function returns. If this problem occurs, the drug must be discontinued until the problem is resolved.

5. **Chronic fatigue.** As mentioned in side effect number one above, amitriptyline can make a patient sleepy. This property is helpful for promoting nighttime sleep and decreasing evening voiding but sometimes the effect seems to last all day; patients just can't function well. There are two factors to consider here. First, it's quite common for amitriptyline to have this effect when a patient is starting out on a course of therapy. It's an effect that can last about two, sometimes three weeks, but gradually subsides. The second possibility is that the dose is too high for the individual and needs to be readjusted down. It's amazing to observe the individual differences in tolerance from patient to patient. Some patients can take 75 or 100 mg and have no fatigue whatsoever, while other patients are terribly lethargic at doses as low as 10 mg per evening. Be careful when mixing amitriptyline with alcoholic beverages or other medications that make you tired— they can have an additive effect.

6. **Weight gain.** Amitriptyline seems to stimulate the appetite and may cause some decrease in the body's metabolism, hence, easy weight gain. Consequently, it's very important to continue an exercise regime and to carefully watch what you eat. Just imagine that every time you pop a cookie into your mouth, your body may be processing it as if you ingested two to three cookies. So be careful.

7. **Decrease in sex drive (libido)/Difficulty achieving orgasm.** These are fairly common problems associated with the tricyclic antidepressants. Lowering the dose or changing the medication to another within this class of medications can be useful but in many cases the problem continues. In such instances, the patient needs to decide whether it's going to be worthwhile to take the drug. The deciding factor is usually the degree of symptom improvement that occurs. Most patients whose symptoms dramatically improve while taking the medication are willing to accept this frustrating side effect. Difficulty achieving orgasm during sexual intercourse is unfortunately a "non-issue" with many patients because the pain associated with orgasm or penile penetration is already precluding sexual encounters.

Other side effects that can occur but are fairly rare include:

1. **Palpitations:** This is the feeling that your heart skipped a beat or that it is fluttering in your chest. If this occurs, the dosage needs to be lowered or the drug discontinued. If you have a history of heart disease, particularly heart arrhythmias, your primary care physician or a cardiologist should be consulted.

2. **Changes in liver function or blood test results:** These problems are extremely uncommon, particularly at the low doses used for the IC patient. Your clinician may want you to take periodic blood tests.

3. **Over-the-counter medication interactions.** Cimetidine (Tagamet®) is a common over-the-counter medication that might interact with tricyclic antidepressants. Cimetidine is commonly used in the treatment of gastritis or stomach ulcer disease. Patients with thyroid disease or a history of narrow angle glaucoma must be monitored closely by their physicians while taking these medications.

Other Tricyclic Antidepressants

Other tricyclic antidepressants frequently used to treat patients with IC include the following:

* Nortriptyline (Pamelor®)

* Doxepin (Sinequan®)

* Imipramine (Tofranil®)

Selective Serotonin Reuptake Inhibitors (SSRIs)

Clinical depression is most commonly treated with these medications because they have fewer side effects than the tricyclic antidepressants. Some clinicians have been using them to treat the symptoms associated with IC. It has been our experience that these medications may help reduce the symptoms of IC but they are usually not as successful at accomplishing this task as the tricyclic antidepressants. There is no published literature establishing a relationship between symptom improvement and treatment with SSRIs in the IC patient.

Examples

* Fluoxetine (Prozac®)   * Sertraline (Zoloft®)

* Paroxetine (Paxil®)   * Citalopram (Celexa®)

* Fluvoxamine (Luvox®)   * Venlafaxine (Effexor®)

Side Effects

Some of the important side effects that need to be considered by the IC patient include the following:

* Nausea in 20–30 percent of patients

* Headache

* Diarrhea. Note that some of these medications are associated with constipation

* Agitation

* Sexual dysfunction. This is one of the most disturbing problems associated with SSRI medications, occurring in up to 50 percent of patients. Difficulties with sexual desire, arousal, and orgasm have been described. If this is bothering you, be sure to discuss it with your doctor. Sometimes changing the medication within this group of medications can partially or totally solve the problem.

* Weight gain or weight loss

Antihistamines

High levels of histamine are found in the bladder walls of many IC patients, hence antihistamines are commonly used in the treatment of interstitial cystitis. Several types of antihistamines have been used, hydroxyzine being the most popular.

Hydroxyzine (Atarax®, Vistaril®)

Hydroxyzine is another medication that can significantly decrease the symptoms of IC. Hydroxyzine is an antihistamine that belongs to the family of medications called H-1 receptor blockers. It prevents the release of histamine, an inflammation-provoking substance released from mast cells (see chapter 3, What Causes Interstitial Cystitis). As you may recall, many patients with IC have increased numbers of these cells in their bladder walls.

Hydroxyzine is given in doses from 10–75 mg at bedtime. It can take anywhere between two weeks to three months to see symptom improvement. The dose of hydroxyzine usually starts at 10–25 mg. Dosage is then slowly increased to 75 mg at night over the course of one month. Hydroxyzine can make you a bit sleepy and therefore, like amitriptyline, can increase the duration of your sleep. It also has some qualities of a muscle relaxant, which is often useful in the treatment of accompanying pelvic floor dysfunction.

Side Effects

There are few side effects associated with hydroxyzine. The biggest problem that we've encountered is fatigue. Many patients complain that they just can't get out of bed the next morning. Like amitriptyline, it's important not to take the medication too late at night (in these circumstances the drug is still circulating at high levels in the bloodstream on waking and therefore fatigue is still present). Sometimes this effect disappears after one to two weeks. Unfortunately, in just as many instances, the fatigue continues. In these cases, it's probably best simply to lower the evening dose or to split the dose into a very low dose (10 mg) in the morning and 10 mg in the evening. In some instances, even smaller doses can be administered by using the liquid form of hydroxyzine. If all else fails, the medication must be discontinued. When symptom relief has been achieved, it's possible either to discontinue or decrease the dose of hydroxyzine. Many patients will continue without any signs of symptom recurrence; however, in just as many patients, symptoms recur. Symptoms can recur within a few days to a few weeks but should disappear again when the medication's original dosage is reinstituted.

Remember, these are only suggestions for use. The final decision of which medication to use and how it is dispensed must be made by your treating clinician.

There are no significant drug interactions associated with hydroxyzine. The most important problem to avoid is excessive lethargy. This can occur by mixing hydroxyzine with other medications that cause fatigue (or alcoholic beverages).

Cromolyn Sodium (Gastrocrom®)

Cromolyn is an anti-inflammatory agent most commonly used to prevent asthmatic attacks and severe nasal allergies. It is also indicated for patients who suffer from mastocytosis, a disease in which mast cells are found in the skin and in other organs. When found in the skin, these cells may release inflammation-causing chemicals (histamine, leukotrienes, etc.), thus causing significant itching. Cromolyn decreases the release of these chemicals and hence, hopefully, reduces symptoms.

As noted in the discussion regarding hydroxyzine, increased numbers of mast cells are found in the bladder walls of many IC patients; and just as with hydroxyzine, some clinicians have treated IC patients with cromolyn. *To date, no studies have been performed to determine the efficacy of this treatment for the IC patient.* The use of cromolyn instillations directly into the bladder has been studied and is discussed in chapter 6, Medications Introduced into the Bladder.

Cromolyn is usually administered as 200 mg taken four times daily, one-half hour before meals and at bedtime. The medication comes as either a liquid concentrate or powder in a gelatin capsule. It needs to be mixed in water before consuming. The dose is continued for several weeks to determine if the patient feels better. If the patient notes fewer symptoms, the medication is usually lowered to the minimum dose needed to keep those symptoms at bay.

Few side effects are associated with oral cromolyn therapy. Diarrhea and headaches are the most frequent problems reported.

Cimetidine (Tagamet)

Cimetidine belongs to a group of medications called H-2 receptor blockers. It was initially developed to decrease stomach acid production in order to treat gastritis (inflammation of the stomach often produced from too much acid secretion) and stomach ulcer disease. Apart from this role, cimetidine has been used as adjunctive therapy in the treatment of hives, a condition caused in large part by the release of histamine from mast cells.

In 1994, a pilot study was performed by Dr. P. Seshadri who treated nine patients with IC with 300 mg of cimetidine twice per day for one month. Six of the nine patients had symptomatic improvement with four of those patients having complete relief of their symptoms. These results are encouraging but due to limited numbers of patients, cimetidine is not considered to be a first-line medication in the treatment of IC.

Although cimetidine is an over-the-counter medication, there are potential interactions with other medications that an IC patient might be taking. For example, cimetidine may cause an increase in the blood levels of diazepam (Valium®), some tricyclic antidepressants, and nifedipine (only the oral solution). Cimetidine shouldn't be taken at the same time as antacids because the antacids can impair proper absorption of the cimetidine. Other drug interactions exist so it's important to notify your physician and pharmacist of all other prescription and nonprescription medications that you're taking. As a final note, another H-2 receptor blocker, ranitidine (Zantac®) is also available over-the-counter. This medication has the same mechanism of action as cimetidine, but has fewer drug interactions. Unfortunately, no clinical studies have been performed to determine ranitidine's efficacy in the treatment of IC.

Antiseizure Medications

Antiseizure medications have been used for many years in the management of neuropathic pain (pain caused by abnormalities in nerve function) with reasonable success. These agents were most popular in the treatment of chronic facial pain and for the pain associated with diabetes. It seems that nerve abnormalities of a similar sort exist in a large number of IC patients. Indeed, those patients often respond favorably to these medications.

Gabapentin (Neurontin®)

Gabapentin is a relatively new medication whose initial use was in the management of seizure disorders. Over the past several years, gabapentin has been found to be useful in the treatment of many diseases associated with pain but it has not received FDA approval for this purpose. Nevertheless this medication has developed an important niche in the field of pain management. Gabapentin is administered as a capsule. It is usually started at low doses, about 100 mg per day but it can go as high as 3600 mg per day in three divided doses. Usually, patients don't need to go to the maximum dose to experience some symptom relief. Gabapentin can be administered along with most other medications used in the treatment of IC. Antacids, however, seem to decrease the blood levels of the medication. It's therefore advised to take gabapentin about two hours after taking an antacid.

One important issue to be concerned about is the fatigue factor. Like amitriptyline and hydroxyzine, gabapentin often causes some sleepiness. This quality is helpful at night but it can be bothersome during the day. When taking multiple medications of this sort, you can end up sleeping all day long and certainly not perform too well at work. Even more important, I don't particularly want to be in the lane next to you while you are driving to work. So be careful! Inform your physician. He or she might need to make some dosage adjustments along the way.

Carbamazepine (Tegretol®)

Like gabapentin, carbamazepine is FDA-approved as an antiseizure medication. Carbamazepine has been a "staple" medication used for patients suffering from chronic pain. It's been well documented to help relieve pain in many patients suffering from trigeminal neuralgia (chronic facial pain) and diabetic neuropathy (pain associated with nerve damage caused by diabetes). We generally don't use these medications as "first-line" therapy but they are frequently helpful with patients who have failed more conventional oral therapy.

Carbamazepine comes in tablet and liquid forms. Generally, the medication is taken twice per day with combined daily doses usually starting at a 200 mg. As a rule, the dose is slowly increased until symptom improvement occurs. Doses can be increased to as high as 1200 mg per day. Your doctor might wish to obtain some initial blood tests and repeat them from time to time. The tests are performed because, though rarely, the medication can affect the production of blood cells or liver function. Some clinicians might want to follow the carbamazepine level in the bloodstream.

The most common side effects include fatigue or dizziness. These effects are usually seen at higher doses. Patients must stop the drug and contact their physician if they develop fever, rashes, or easy bruising. Interstitial cystitis patients need to be careful to avoid interactions with other drugs that might be prescribed to treat their bladder condition such as cimetidine and calcium channel blockers (like nifedipine). Also, keep in mind that carbamazepine might worsen the fatigue effect from other medications or alcohol.

Non-Steroidal Anti-Inflammatory Medications (NSAIDs)

NSAIDs are medications that have been traditionally used for mild to moderate pain. They appear to work by decreasing prostaglandin release in our bodies. Prostaglandins are chemicals that stimulate inflammation. The most well-known NSAID medication is aspirin. The one big drawback of these medications is their effect on the stomach lining. Most have a tendency to cause stomach upset and in the worst setting, actually cause gastritis or stomach ulcers. In an attempt to avoid this problem, patients are always cautioned to take these medications with food. Recently, a new group of these medications has been developed that has less potential for causing stomach problems. These are the cox-2 inhibitors (Celebrex® and Vioxx®). Keep in mind that they can still cause stomach upset.

Examples

* Acetosalicylic acid (Aspirin)

* Ibuprofen (Motrin®)

* Piroxicam (Feldene®)

* Naproxen (Naprosyn®)

* Indomethacin (Indocin®)

* Celecoxib (Celebrex)

* Rofecoxib (Vioxx)

Immunosuppressants

Autoimmune diseases are occasionally seen in the IC patient. Immunosuppressants (medications that decrease the efficiency of your immune system) are often used in the treatment of these conditions. They are rarely used in the IC patient without an obvious autoimmune disease, due to their numerous and potentially devastating side effects.

Steroids

The most common immunosuppressant used in medical practice is prednisone. Prednisone is part of a class of medications (and hormones) called steroids. Published reports (Badenoch 1971) suggest that prednisone and similar medications can decrease the symptoms in IC patients in as many as 76 percent of patients. But—and there's a *big* but here—most clinicians who routinely treat IC patients are reluctant to place their patients on this therapy. The major reason that we shy away from this therapy relates to the potential complications associated with steroid administration. Some problems that we particularly worry about are as follows:

1. The development of osteoporosis (calcium loss from bones leading to easy fractures)

2. Increased susceptibility to infection

3. Worsening of any diabetes, if present, or the development of diabetes while taking the steroids

4. Fluid retention

5. Weight gain

6. Increased bruisability

7. Aseptic necrosis of the femoral head. This complication causes the upper part of the patient's thigh bone to die, leading to pain and severe arthritis in this region

8. Many relapses were observed after the initial 76 percent improvement rate (Badenoch 1971) initially seen with prednisone therapy

9. The dose of steroid therapy is usually administered over two to three months

10. The dose is relatively high. Prednisone is usually administered at a starting dose of 15 mg each day and is tapered down to a dose of 5 mg each day

Many more problems related to steroid use are seen but they usually occur with therapy that's given for longer than two to three months (the usual length of time that predisone is administered to IC patients).

Other problems that occur include the frequent relapses when therapy is discontinued. Overall, the potential risks associated with steroid use versus the potential benefits derived from these medications suggest that we should hold off with their use unless absolutely necessary. As you'll see in chapter 6, instilling steroids directly into the bladder is probably a much better strategy since there's little absorption into the bloodstream by that route.

Muscle Relaxants

A great deal of pelvic floor muscle spasticity often accompanies interstitial cystitis. Furthermore, muscle spasms that occur with associated fibromyalgia can worsen a seemingly impossible to worsen disease (see the section in chapter 4, "Pelvic Floor Dysfunction"). Muscle relaxants, along with appropriate conservative therapy is usually tremendously helpful in the treatment of these frequent problems.

Diazepam (Valium)

Valium is a member of a family of medications called the benzodiazepines. They became popularized for the treatment of anxiety-related disorders in the 1960s and have since been found to be useful in the treatment of seizure disorders and muscle spasm. Diazepam is most frequently prescribed for the IC patient to treat associated pelvic floor dysfunction. Other benzodiazepines are available but little literature is available on their role in muscle spasticity syndromes.

The dose of diazepam in the treatment of pelvic floor dysfunction is usually 2 mg three times daily. When symptoms have decreased, patients are encouraged to slowly reduce the dose with the ultimate hope of taking the medication only on an "as needed" basis.

Diazepam received a bad rap in the media in the 1970s and 1980s. Some patients began abusing the medication, taking it as a recreational drug. These patients were taking high doses of the diazepam to become euphoric. When diazepam is prescribed properly in low doses, euphoria should never occur. *The benzodiazepines have not been associated with psychotic behavior, hallucinations, or delusions.* Physical dependence (meaning that a withdrawal syndrome can occur with abrupt cessation of the medication) may take place with benzodiazepines; however, with low dose therapy, this is a rare event. When it does occur, withdrawal may manifest as sensitivity to light and sound, tremulousness, or insomnia. These problems are generally not very severe and are self-limited.

Side Effects

The major side effects of the benzodiazepines include the following:

1. **Fatigue.** This is usually not a big problem when administering low doses of these medicines. When it does occur, it usually slowly disappears within the first few weeks of therapy. On the other hand, some patients are very sensitive to medications; that is, they are much more profoundly affected by the medication than one would anticipate. If you are that type of patient, it's probably best to start off with one-half of a tablet taken three times per day. Keep in mind that the major goal of therapy is to have symptom improvement while one is not aware that the medication is working.

   Be careful when mixing diazepam with alcohol or other medications that can cause fatigue. You may have no apparent side effects while taking a low dose of diazepam; however, let's say that your physician prescribes a low dose of amitriptyline along with the diazepam. Either of these doses alone might not be associated with a great deal of lethargy but combining them together can sometimes be a problem. The solution is to see how your body reacts to taking them together. *This is not the time to take a long car drive at night on a wet and curvy road.* If you have no problem, that's great. If you experience some fatigue, this sometimes abates as you continue to take your medications. Sometimes, though, the fatigue does continue. In that case, it warrants either changing the doses or discontinuing one of the medications.

2. **Depression.** Patients who are being treated for depression can have a worsening of their depression during treatment with the benzodiazepines. Taking low doses of diazepam is usually not a problem in the face of depression; however, if you feel as though your depression is worsening, relay this information to your physician. The physician will then usually discontinue the medication. Rarely, patients who have had no history of depression do report a problem with depression while being treated with benzodiazepines. This is another instance where the medication is usually discontinued.

3. **Unusual reactions.** Although the benzodiazepines are well-known for their calming effect, a rare patient will report the opposite effect. In these situations, patients report a feeling of hostility or anger. Instead of having a good night's sleep, they report sleeping very poorly. This is another instance where the drug is usually discontinued.

Other Muscle Relaxants

Other commonly used muscle relaxants include:

* Baclofen (Lioresal®)

* Methocarbamol (Robaxin®)

* Cyclobenzaprine (Flexeril®)

* Orphenadrine (Norflex®)

* Metaxalone (Skelaxin®)

* Carisoprodol (Soma®)

* Chlorzoxazone (Paraflex®/Parafon Forte®)

* Chlorphenesin carbamate (Maloate®)

None of these agents has stood out as clearly superior within the group. They all have similar side effects. These include lethargy, dizziness, headaches, and blurred vision. Medication abuse is uncommon but has been reported with long-term use.

Narcotic Therapy

Narcotics, also called opioids, are medications that can significantly reduce pain. They are most commonly prescribed for the management of acute (short-lived) pain. Common situations where narcotics are used include the following:

1. Management of post-operative pain

2. Management of pain that will probably subside within hours to weeks. A common example of this pain is that which often arises with kidney stones. In this scenario, the patient might come into the emergency room with excruciating pain as the stone is passing through the urinary tract. The pain subsides somewhat. The doctors in the emergency room send the patient home hoping that the stone will pass within a short time. Narcotics are prescribed for the patient to take should the pain return. The doctors don't expect the patient to be taking the narcotics for a very long time and don't prescribe more than a week or two's worth of pills.

You may have noticed that no mention has been made thus far of narcotic therapy for the patient who suffers from chronic pain. Unfortunately, this is an area where the medical profession has "traditionally" provided suboptimal service due to unsubstantiated fears of patient drug abuse, dependency, addiction, or medical complications. These fears have led many physicians to treat only terminally ill patients with "liberal" doses of narcotics. Often, when physicians treat patients with diseases such as IC, narcotics are either not offered or patients are underdosed.

Let's take a look at the major concerns that both patients and physicians have regarding narcotic therapy:

1. **Drug abuse.** This is the use of a medication for nonmedical purposes. The concern here is that the patient will use the medicine not just to decrease pain, but to "escape" from life's problems. The patient needs to understand up front that these medications are used to help him/her return to a full life, not to avoid it. It's sometimes difficult for the

physician to determine whether drug abuse is occurring. For example, a patient might ask for higher doses of narcotics for pain relief. Is the patient abusing the medication or is *tolerance* (the need to administer higher doses of a medication to achieve the same effect) taking place? This can be a tough one to answer, even for the patient. Probably the best way to differentiate between these two problems is for the physician to look at what's going on in the patient's life. We would expect the patient's mood, job status, and family life to be slowly improving if the narcotics are serving their intended function. Consultation with family members can be a helpful unbiased resource when narcotic abuse is a consideration.

2. **Drug addiction.** Drug addiction is a compulsive pattern of drug abuse associated with socially inappropriate or dangerous behaviors. This is a psychiatric illness that is not caused by narcotics. Addiction is an extremely rare event in patients who have chronic pain. Nevertheless, this is the most common reason that patients decline narcotic therapy (and that doctors withhold it). There is the fear that the patient might "turn into an addict." Actually, patients who are worried about that issue probably have the lowest risk of all of becoming addicted to narcotics.

3. **Pseudoaddiction.** This term was coined to describe the patient who is preoccupied with obtaining his or her narcotic and who increases the dose without physician approval—but in this case the patient is not abusing the medication; neither does the patient have an addiction. Rather, the patient is still in pain despite the prescribed dose of narcotic. Instead of relaying this information to the caregiver, the patient takes it upon himself/herself to dose appropriately. This unsanctioned dosing gives the impression of addiction to many clinicians. The patient is then labeled an "addict" when this simply is not the case. Obviously, this can have a catastrophic effect on the doctor-patient relationship.

4. **Catastrophic medical complications.** In high doses narcotics can cause respiratory depression (a decrease in the "drive" to breathe). Physicians are concerned that patients in pain might take more pills than prescribed to deal with increases in pain, leading to respiratory arrest and death. Slowly increasing the dose of the narcotic to achieve its desired effect prevents this complication from occurring. As you can

imagine, this is a big concern for any patient who abuses his/her medication.

5. **Physical dependency.** Physical dependency is a characteristic of all narcotics. This means that the sudden cessation or reduction in narcotic dose will often result in physical illness (the withdrawal syndrome). It occurs most frequently in patients who have been on narcotic therapy for long periods of time. This problem can usually be avoided by slowly reducing (tapering) the dose.

On the bright side, over the past ten years many physicians have been much more willing to dispense long-term narcotic therapy to patients with nonterminally ill patient's pain. Although many primary care physicians and specialists will dispense narcotics in these situations, some still feel uncomfortable managing problems such as physical dependency, which occur more frequently at higher doses. In these situations, pain management specialists can be helpful. These are physicians (usually neurologists or anesthesiologists) who have made a new niche for themselves on the medical scene and are probably the best resource for patients and their clinicians regarding narcotic therapy, particularly when fairly high doses of narcotics are needed for pain control.

Now comes the most important question: Which patients should be receiving narcotic therapy? Many factors must be considered such as the patient's age, other prescribed medications, other medical illnesses, the severity of the pain, and the patient's response to previous pain management. As a general principle, narcotics are dispensed on a chronic basis when other medical therapies cannot adequately relieve the patient's discomfort. Narcotics are frequently used early on in therapy in those patients who present with unremitting severe pain. Once the pain has subsided a bit, other medical therapy can be administered while the narcotic dosage is lowered or, hopefully, discontinued.

Detailing all of the narcotic preparations available on the market is beyond the scope of this book. These medications can be classified into categories based upon their duration of action (short- or long-acting narcotics) or by their strength (weak versus strong narcotics). Narcotics can be administered as pills, sublingual tablets (the medication is placed under the tongue like a nitroglycerine tablet), rectal suppositories, skin patches, injections, or through an intravenous route. Selecting the proper dose is always done on a case-by-case basis. The type of narcotic prescribed or its dose is changed as the patient's complaints of pain change.

Short- and Long-Acting Narcotic Therapy

When treating with narcotics, the duration of drug action is a very important consideration. Short-acting, long-acting, or combination therapy is administered depending upon the patient's description of pain. For example, let's take a situation where a patient has pain well controlled with a combination of pentosanpolysulfate sodium and amitriptyline, but is having severe pain each morning lasting about four hours. Supplemental narcotic therapy might be considered in this situation. A long-acting narcotic would be inappropriate in this case because the medication would still be at high levels in the bloodstream many hours after the pain dissipated—it exposes the patient to unneeded side effects.

Now to turn the situation around, consider the patient who has unremitting pelvic pain that is unresponsive to other oral medications. Treating this patient with short-acting agents might not achieve the best results. Patients often feel much better fifteen to thirty minutes after taking their medication but may have pain return prior to the next dose. The patient feels better but he or she would probably benefit even more by being placed on a long-acting narcotic. "Transdermal" skin patches are an alternative way to administer narcotics over a long period of time. These patches, when applied to the skin, allow the narcotic dose to be reliably absorbed through the skin and permit a steady, constant infusion of the medication into the bloodstream.

Finally, some patients benefit greatly from a combination of short- and long-acting narcotics. Those are patients who have chronic moderate to severe pain but whose pain "goes through the roof" for relatively short intervals. Those patients may benefit from taking a long-acting narcotic to manage the chronic moderate pain, supplemented by a short-acting narcotic to be used when the pain intermittently escalates. In the hospital setting, it's a lot easier to take care of these problems due to techniques like "patient-controlled anesthesia" or PCA. With PCA, the patient has an intravenous line in place and a button at the bedside. A constant low level of narcotic is administered via the IV drip; but if the patient suddenly feels that the pain is increasing, he or she can press the button, which then allows an extra dose of narcotic to be administered. A very interesting advance in medical technology that may be able to provide therapy akin to PCA—but at home—is a transdermal skin patch that allows the patient to have both long- and short-acting therapy. This patch will provide a constant dose of narcotic, but when pain intensifies, the patient will have the opportunity to press a small "button" on the patch. This button creates a small electrical charge on the skin (it doesn't hurt) that allows a "pulse" of extra medication to be administered. This device is currently under development and is not yet available.

Strong and Weak Narcotic Therapy

There exists a wide range of potencies amongst the various narcotics. This is an important issue to consider when the physician selects an agent. The physician gauges which narcotic to administer based upon symptom severity. Patients who are in severe pain should be given high potency narcotics first, rather than starting out with inevitably unsuccessful weak medications. In the most severe circumstances, patients need to be admitted to the hospital to receive strong narcotics by injection or by an intravenous route.

Side Effects Associated with Narcotic Therapy

Apart from problems associated with medication misuse, narcotics can have side effects, just as any other medication can. The major side effects to be concerned about include the following:

1. **Constipation.** This is the most common adverse reaction seen with narcotic therapy. Unlike many side effects of narcotics that subside or disappear with continued usage, constipation usually persists. This is an important consideration when starting an IC patient on narcotics. Constipation is a frequent problem seen in IC patients and can, all by itself, cause a worsening of pelvic pain and urgency/frequency of urination. It's therefore important to treat constipation very aggressively, hopefully even before the narcotics are taken. Laxatives and/or stool softeners are often prescribed on a daily or as needed basis to deal with this problem. Common laxatives used include Milk of Magnesia, senna (Senokot®), lactulose, and magnesium citrate.

2. **Nausea and Vomiting.** These problems occur in about 25–30 percent of patients, particularly as the doses are escalating. Fortunately, the nausea usually lessens in severity or disappears within a few weeks. Nausea can develop for three reasons. First, as noted in number one, narcotics slow down the functioning of the intestines and the stomach. This can lead to a bloating sensation caused by a "back up" of

stomach and intestinal contents. Patients usually develop this bloating shortly after a meal. Patients may also note the sensation of early fullness. The clinician will sometimes treat this problem with metoclopramide (Reglan®), a medication that speeds up stomach emptying. It's also important to treat any associated constipation.

A second cause of nausea is the narcotic's effect on our sense of balance. Many patients note that their nausea is associated with some dizziness or is induced by motion. When this occurs, prochlorperazine (Compazine®), scopolamine (Transderm Scop®), or meclizine (Antivert®) may be helpful.

The third cause of nausea is the narcotic's direct effect on nausea-triggering centers in the brain. Medications that have been used to treat this problem include prochlorperazine (Compazine®) or metoclopramide (Reglan). Hydroxyzine, a "staple" medication used in the management of IC (see above), can also decrease nausea.

3. **Sedation.** This is another side effect of narcotic administration that usually settles down within a few days to weeks. Stimulants are occasionally administered to patients who absolutely need their narcotic dose but whose lethargy persists despite drug or dose changes.

4. **Confusion.** Mild confusion occasionally occurs when narcotic doses are increased. The effect is usually temporary but if the problem persists alternative medications are considered. Delirium, an agitated state marked by confusion and sometimes hallucinations and delusions, is rare. When it occurs, delirium is usually seen in elderly or debilitated patients.

5. **Urinary retention.** Narcotics can affect bladder function. They decrease the force of a bladder contraction and, hence, some patients will notice a decrease in the force of their urinary stream. The problem can be so severe as to require placement of a temporary catheter in the bladder to allow the urine to pass. Patients who are more susceptible to this side effect are those men whose urine flow is already a bit slow from enlargement of the prostate or those men and women with pelvic floor dysfunction. Patients who are starting therapy with a narcotic but who are already taking medications that can slow bladder function (such as Elavil, Ditropan®, Detrol®) should watch out for a worsening of this problem.

6. **Respiratory depression.** Respiratory depression is a potentially deadly complication of narcotic therapy but, fortunately, this side effect is rare and is usually encountered only when administering high doses of narcotics. Elderly or debilitated patients appear to be more susceptible to this problem. Usually increased fatigue or confusion precedes this respiratory problem. As discussed above, changes in the type of narcotic prescribed or dosage changes may be necessary as the level of pain changes. This is extremely important for all IC patients whose pain typically waxes and wanes. This relates to problems with respiratory depression as follows: Suppose an IC patient is taking a high dose of a narcotic on a chronic basis for pain. The patient undergoes several instillations of DMSO (see chapter 6, Medications Introduced into the Bladder) and the pain improves greatly. This decrease in pain in the face of continued high doses of narcotic (now beyond the dose needed for adequate pain relief) may result in severe fatigue, confusion, and respiratory depression.

"Atypical" Opioids

The term "atypical opioids" implies that these agents can be technically classified as narcotics but don't appear to have many of the "typical" side effects of the opioids. In this sense, these medications are safer than most narcotics. Unfortunately, they are usually somewhat less potent. They work best in the treatment of mild to moderate pain.

Tramadol (Ultram)

Tramadol hydrocholride has been useful in the management of moderate pain. Based upon its mechanism of action, tramadol is a narcotic but it lacks many of the typical side effects associated with narcotics. Specifically, unlike that group of medications, tramadol doesn't seem to have any effect on one's drive to breathe (it doesn't cause respiratory depression) nor does it usually cause significant problems with constipation. Furthermore, there doesn't seem to be a big problem with drug tolerance (needing higher and higher doses of the medication to achieve the same pain-relieving effect).

As stated above, tramadol is helpful for pain that is moderate in severity. It is most commonly administered as a 50 mg tablet but higher strengths are available. Tramadol is taken as 1–2 tablets every four to six hours and is used only when pain is present. Pain relief usually begins about one hour after the dose is taken. Maximum pain relief occurs about two to three hours after the dose. Patients are told not to take more than 400 mg per day. The most commonly encountered side effects include fatigue, nausea, and headache. Because it can make you tired, it's important to be careful when taking this medication with other medications that can cause the same problem (such as hydroxyzine or amitriptyline).

Urinary Anesthetics

These are medications which, when taken orally, are excreted into the urine and may decrease the sensitivity of the bladder and urethral lining. They are often dispensed in the face of a urinary tract infection, a condition where significant urethral burning with urination is encountered. Overall, the medications are only occasionally useful in decreasing the symptoms of IC.

Phenazopyridine Hydrochloride (Pyridium®)

Phenazopyridine is a urinary anesthetic that turns the urine a bright orange color. This medication is often prescribed to decrease the urethral burning associated with procedures such as catheterization or cystoscopy. Phenazopyridine is also commonly administered to decrease burning associated with urinary tract infections. The usual dose is 100–200 mg taken three times per day.

Phenazopyridine usually doesn't help relieve the symptoms of IC (although here and there a patient will have symptom improvement) but can be helpful when invasive procedures are performed. The biggest problem associated with this medication is its ability to stain everything in sight. It's therefore not a great drug to use when the entire house and all the bathroom(s) are carpeted white. This medication is not recommended for long-term use because of its potential to affect the production of blood cells in the bone marrow.

Atropine Sulfate, Benzoic Acid, Hyoscyamine, Methenamine, Methylene Blue, Phenyl Salicylate (Urised®)

Urised is a "combination" medication. It contains a urinary anesthetic (similar in that respect to pyridium), a urinary antiseptic (kills bacteria), and an anticholinergic agent (relaxes the bladder). Let's look at these components separately.

* **Methenamine.** This medication, when exposed to relatively acid urine, is converted to formaldehyde. Formaldehyde then kills bacteria. You may be thinking right now, "Formaldehyde! Isn't that the 'pickling' solution used to preserve cadavers?" The answer is, you bet it is; but the dose is so low, it doesn't affect the bladder surface at all.

* **Methylene blue and benzoic acid:** These medications also help to kill bacteria in the urine. The methylene blue turns the urine a blue color. The benzoic acid helps acidify the urine, thus enhancing the effect of the methenamine.

* **Phenyl salicylate:** This agent is a mild analgesic.

* **Atropine sulfate and hyoscyamine:** Both of these medications relax the bladder and inhibit unwanted bladder contractions.

The usual dose of Urised is two tablets four times per day when it's used to treat urinary tract infections. The medication is often used to prevent infections from occurring or to treat symptoms of urinary urgency, frequency, or burning. When the medication is given in that capacity it may be administered in lower doses such as two tablets two to three times per day.

Side effects, when they occur, are usually mild. The side effects are usually related to the anticholinergic portion of the medication, the atropine sulfate and hyoscyamine.

Anticholinergic Therapy

The majority of the bladder wall is composed of muscle. That's important because the muscle of the bladder must contract in order to urinate properly. Anticholinergic medications slow down bladder function and can, therefore, be useful for those patients who have bladders that contract when they are not supposed to (this condition is also called "overactive bladder" or "bladder instability"). Most patients who have interstitial cystitis have an over*sensitive* bladder, not an overactive bladder. Nevertheless, it's thought that as many as 10 percent of IC patients have some degree of bladder overactivity, so a trial of these medications may be offered to patients. Anticholinergic agents that you might encounter include the following:

* Oxybutinin (Ditropan, Ditropan XL®). This is one of the most widely used anticholinergic medications. Oxybutinin is available in generic form. It is usually given in doses of 2.5–5mg two to three times daily. The drug can also be administered on an as needed basis. Ditropan XL is a newly

released form of oxybutinin that is a once-a-day tablet. A constant release of the medication occurs during the day that may result in fewer side effects and better efficacy. Another advantage of this preparation is that the tablet itself is inert. The tablet shell is passed out in the stool while the medication is absorbed. This point is brought up because many IC patients seem to have problems with the gelatin coating used in the "packaging" of many pills and capsules.

1. **Hyoscyamine sulfate (Levbid®, Levsin SL®).** Levbid is an anticholinergic medication administered on a twice-daily basis. Levsin SL is a sublingual (placed under the tongue) tablet that works rapidly to calm down abnormal bladder contractions. It accomplishes this task by being rapidly absorbed in the bloodstream. One to two tablets of Levsin SL can be taken every four to six hours as needed.

2. **Tolterodine (Detrol).** Detrol is a recently introduced anticholinergic agent. It is administered on a twice-daily basis. It appears to be associated with fewer side effects such as dry mouth and constipation.

3. **Tricyclic antidepressants.** These medications vary in their anticholinergic effects. In some patients, these effects may help to improve patient's symptoms. However, the anticholinergic effects often limit the dose of medication that can be used.

Side Effects

1. **Constipation.** Anticholinergic medications are well-known to slow down the function of the bladder and the intestines. Slowing down the intestines can lead to constipation. This quality can actually be helpful to a patient who suffers from intermittent bouts of diarrhea. It's very important to deal with the constipation with diet changes or stool softeners/laxatives as needed *before* thinking about anticholinergic therapy. If constipation becomes a problem during therapy, changes can be made in the medication or the dosage.

2. **Dry mouth.** This is the most common problem associated with anticholinergic therapy. It occurs because anticholinergic medications decrease the amount of saliva produced in the salivary glands. As you can imagine, this can be a very disturbing problem. Some patients find that keeping sucking candy nearby is helpful. Many patients carry a water bottle around at all times and take small sips throughout the day.

Biotene mouthwash, toothpaste, and dental chewing gum were formulated by Laclede Professional Products, Inc. (800-922-5856 or www.laclede.com) to help soothe complaints of dry mouth. The company also manufactures a moisturizing gel that functions as an artificial saliva for eight hours. These are products that can be purchased over the counter at most drug stores.

3. **Lethargy.** This is a relatively uncommon problem seen with this group of medicines but, in some instances, severe fatigue can necessitate discontinuing therapy.

4. **Eye pain.** Anticholinergic medications should not be administered to patients with a condition called "narrow angle glaucoma." Most patients who have glaucoma have "open angle glaucoma." If you have glaucoma but are uncertain of the type that you have, make sure to call your ophthalmologist before starting therapy. For patients with narrow angle glaucoma, taking anticholinergic medications can cause high pressures to develop within the eye, causing a permanent worsening of vision.

L-arginine

Before discussing the role of L-arginine in interstitial cystitis, it's important to have a basic knowledge about nitric oxide (NO). Nitric oxide is a gas that is produced in our bodies and has an important role in the following functions:

* Killing bacteria

* Killing tumor cells

* Facilitating smooth muscle relaxation (this is the type of muscle found in the bladder)

* Transmitting pain within nerves

* Releasing hormones

* Modulating the immune system

Nitric oxide is a very hot research topic these days with much attention being paid to its role in the urinary tract. Nitric oxide research as it relates to interstitial cystitis is just beginning to develop and as frequently happens with new research endeavors, there's controversy and conflicting data. Ehren, Hosseini, Lundberg, and Wiklund (1999) demonstrated that two sets of patients, those with bladder infections and those suffering from IC (only eight patients were evaluated), had high bladder NO levels. In contrast, studies at Yale University (Smith, Wheeler, Foster, Jr., and Weiss 1996) have shown IC patients to have reduced quantities of nitric oxide synthase (a chemical that also helps to create nitric oxide) in their urine, suggesting that NO levels in IC patients are low. The question then arises, would it be helpful to the IC patient to increase the level of NO in the bladder or decrease it? There is experimental evidence that suggests that either of these approaches might improve symptoms. The group at Yale decided to increase NO levels (since their previous studies suggested low levels of bladder NO in IC) by administering L-arginine (Smith, Wheeler, Foster, Jr., and Weiss 1997).

Amino acids are the "building blocks" of proteins. L-arginine is an amino acid that is involved in the production of nitric oxide. L-arginine itself may play a role in the production of naturally produced analgesic chemicals in the body. The Yale study showed, by administering 1.5 grams of L-arginine per day for six months to eight patients, that the levels of nitric oxide synthase were increased. More importantly, they followed ten patients who received the same therapy and noted "significant" decreases in lower abdominal pain, urethral/vaginal pain, and urinary frequency within one month of starting therapy. Lower abdominal pain decreased from an average of 5.0 (on a 0–10 pain scale, 0 indicating no pain and 10 indicating the most severe pain) to 1.5 after six months. Vaginal/urethral pain decreased from a score of 4.5 to 1.5. Nighttime urination decreased from an average of 5.3 bathroom visits to 1.9.

This sounded pretty good, but follow-up studies weren't quite as impressive. Ehren, Hosseini, Lundberg, and Wiklund (1998) reported their results when administering relatively high doses of L-arginine (3 or 10 grams per day) to IC patients for five weeks. They found no significant change in bladder NO levels nor did they find any change in overall IC symptoms. The group from Yale (Korting, Smith, Wheeler, and Weiss 1999) performed a double-blind placebo-controlled trial (patients and their doctors were not allowed to know whether the patients were taking the "real" medication or a "sugar pill" until the study was completed) in fifty-three IC patients. Daytime frequency didn't change much from an average of 13.6 voids at the beginning of the study to 14.3 at three months. Nighttime voids also averaged 3.0 at the beginning and 2.9 at the end of the study. There were no significant decreases in overall symptom scores at three months. Interestingly, these researchers examined several patients within the study group who *did* have significant symptom improvement on the L-arginine. These patients tended to have a history of intermittent urinary tract infections and higher bladder capacities (greater than 800 cc).

Our experience with L-arginine in IC patients has been rather disappointing; however, there seems to be no harm in trying this form of therapy for a few months. If the Yale group's findings hold true, patients with high bladder capacities or a history of recurrent urinary tract infections will have a better chance at obtaining symptom improvement. Outside the realm of interstitial cystitis, research is presently being conducted to evaluate the potential role of nitric oxide synthase inhibitors in pain reduction. So far, the results are encouraging. It will probably be a few years before any of these medications are commercially available.

Calcium Channel Blockers

Calcium channel blockers are medications that have been traditionally used to treat angina (chest pain related to the heart) and high blood pressure. These medications are known to relax smooth muscle (the type of muscle found in the bladder) and to inhibit certain types of inflammation.

Nifedipine (Procardia®, Procardia XL®)

Nifedipine is a calcium channel blocker that has been useful in the treatment of pain associated with a condition called reflex sympathetic dystrophy (RSD). In RSD, changes in the nervous system cause a decrease in blood flow to the limbs. This leads to pain and atrophy (wasting away) of the limb. The bladders of some patients with interstitial cystitis have some of these characteristics (see chapter 3, What Causes Interstitial Cystitis?).

In 1991, Fleischmann, Huntley, Singleton, and Wentworth evaluated the role of nifedipine (at a dose of 30 mg per day) in ten female IC patients. The dose used was 30 mg per day but a few patients needed their dose to be increased to 60 mg per day. Of nine patients who were followed over four months, five patients showed at least a 50 percent decrease in symptoms. Improvement in pain was the first notable effect, followed by a decrease in urinary urgency. Nighttime and daytime urinary frequency didn't change significantly. There are no other clinical studies regarding nifedipine's use in interstitial cystitis.

Procardia XL is the extended release form of this medication and is taken every 24 hours. It's probably the best form of nifedipine to take since it provides a more stable blood level of the drug.

Side Effects

Our use of nifedipine has been hampered by the associated side effects of the medication, far more than noted in the above study. The major side effects of nifedipine include: leg swelling (10 percent), an abnormally low blood pressure (5 percent), fatigue (10 percent), dizziness (10 percent), palpitations (2 percent), and constipation (2 percent). These side effects and reports of unimpressive symptom improvement by most IC patients limited the usefulness of this medication.

Alpha-blockers

Alpha-blockers are medications that were originally designed to decrease blood pressure. The way that they accomplish this task is by causing muscles found in the walls of arteries to relax. Interestingly, the same type of muscle is present in the region of the bladder neck (the region of the bladder where the urine exits) and in the prostate gland.

Examples

* Doxazacin (Cardura®)

* Terazosin (Hytrin®)

* Tamsulosin (Flomax®)

The muscle relaxation in the region of the bladder neck and the prostate gland caused by alpha blockers was found to be incredibly useful to men suffering from urinary symptoms related to the prostate's blockage of urine flow. It appeared that relaxation of the specialized muscle in this region (called "smooth muscle") significantly improved the force of the urine stream for many patients. Subsequently, the pharmaceutical companies that produced these drugs acquired FDA approval for their use in the treatment of "benign prostatic hyperplasia" (the normal growth of the prostate with aging that sometimes blocks the flow of urine). Most male patients who ultimately are diagnosed with IC have had a trial of alpha-blocker therapy in their travels through the medical system. Some of these men have experienced mild symptom improvement on the medication.

Now comes the controversial part. It seems that these medications also can be helpful to some women who suffer from a poor urinary stream and/or who have "urethral pain." Many IC patients have a poor force of their urinary stream. This can be caused by factors such as pelvic floor muscle spasm or to the fact that the flow is often poor when voiding very low volumes of urine. Occasionally, the poor force of the urine stream stems from overtightening of the bladder neck muscles. Unlike the muscles of the pelvic floor, the patient has no ability to relax or contract these muscles. Many clinicians who deal with female patients suffering from a poor force of the urine stream will empirically begin a trial of an alpha-blocker. As mentioned earlier, this is routine care for the male patient but is unconventional therapy for the female (the medications are only FDA-approved for men suffering from prostatic enlargement). If there is improvement in the urine flow or pain, the medication is continued. If not, it's stopped.

Three major alpha-blockers are used in practice today. The first two, doxazocin and terazosin, were originally used to treat high blood pressure. A significant decrease in blood pressure is rarely seen in patients who begin therapy with a blood pressure in the normal range. Nevertheless, dizziness, fatigue, and in very rare instances, fainting (especially with the first dose) can occur. These medications are, therefore, always started at a low dose and are taken just before sleep. Nasal congestion is another common complaint. The dose of the medication is increased, assuming that there are no adverse reactions. The doses of terazosin can range from 1–10 mg at bedtime. At the time of this writing, terazosin, a generic form of terazocin, has just become available. The doses of doxazocin can range from 2–8 mg at bedtime.

Tamsulosin is another alpha-blocker that is more "selective" in terms of its effect on smooth muscle. It appears that this agent relaxes the neck of the bladder wall but doesn't have as much of an effect on muscle within the arteries. Hence, there is little effect on blood pressure. Dizziness and fatigue can occur but are less common than with the other alpha-blockers. It, therefore, doesn't have to be taken at bedtime. As seen with doxazocin and terazosin, nasal congestion can occur. Male patients often complain of a "dry orgasm" (they orgasm but no semen comes out) associated with the alpha-blockers but this appears to be more common with tamsulosin. During orgasm, semen enters the urethra at the level of the prostate. At that time, the neck of the bladder is normally closed off. Muscles contract that propel the semen out through the penis. When you are taking an alpha-blocker, the bladder neck is often relaxed. Hence, when the semen enters the urethra, it takes the path of least resistance back into the bladder. Ejaculation occurs but in the reverse direction, a process called "retrograde ejaculation." Normal ejaculation occurs when the drug is stopped. The dose of tamsulosin ranges from 0.4–0.8 mg per day.

Chapter 6

Medications Introduced into the Bladder

A more direct treatment approach than oral therapy is to instill (to introduce slowly) a medication or combination of medications directly into the bladder. This is called *intravesical therapy* or *intravesical instillation* ("vesical" means bladder). The medications are instilled into the bladder using a catheter, usually on a weekly basis for varying durations—usually twenty to thirty minutes, if possible. Lots of different medications have been placed into patients' bladders in past years. These medications will be reviewed in this chapter, but more time will be spent reviewing those medications that are most commonly used in practice today.

Catheters

Before reviewing the medications that have been instilled into the bladder let's have a word about catheters. The insertion of a urinary catheter is one of the most common procedures used in medical practice. It's usually done either to drain urine from a bladder that's not emptying well or to closely monitor how much urine is being produced over a given period of time (the *urine output*). Although it's very simple to instill medication(s) into a patient's bladder, not many clinicians apart from urologists and some gynecologists routinely perform this sort of therapy.

If you've never been catheterized before, the thought of this tube being placed in your urethra could stir up some pretty nasty images. Men, in particular, are not generally very pleased with this idea. Also, patients who have some degree of preexisting urethral pain usually are very nervous about having the catheter placed. So—what should you expect?

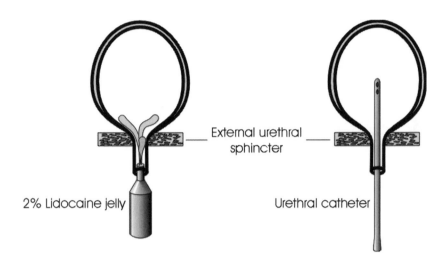

External urethral
sphincter

2% Lidocaine jelly

Urethral catheter

Figure 8. Introducing an anesthetic jelly into the urethra prior to insertion of the Foley catheter.

Prior to placing a catheter many if not most clinicians will instill a water-based lubricant into the urethra. This allows the catheter to slide in with ease. The lubricant often will contain an anesthetic called lidocaine (2 percent lidocaine jelly). Usually, this "anesthetic jelly" is introduced into the urethra through a small cone tip at the end of the dispensing tube (see figure 8). At first you might feel some mild to moderate burning and pressure at the opening of the urethra (the opening is also called the *meatus*). The catheter is then advanced into the bladder. Generally, this proceeds without any difficulty. The most discomfort you might sense occurs when the catheter is being passed beyond the region of the external urinary sphincter. Most IC patients have some associated spasticity of these muscles. When the catheter is passed into this region, many patients (not just IC patients) tend to reflexively tighten these muscles. If the muscles are pulled tight when the catheter passes, the patient will experience discomfort. This is usually perceived as a "pressure-like" pain that is not remedied by the previously administered anesthetic.

At this point the clinician may ask you to "relax" (of course that's easy for them to say!). What is meant by asking you "to relax" is to try to loosen those muscles—don't bear down. Instead, close your eyes, keep your head down on the exam table (lifting it up tends to make you strain even further), and pretend that you're urinating. You won't release urine because the catheter will prevent urine leakage from taking place. This is a pretty helpful maneuver because during the normal process of voiding, one normally relaxes those muscles. Once the catheter is in the bladder, most patients feel much better. Although this process may still sound unnerving to you, the bright side is that it's over in several seconds.

Just the process of catheterization can sometimes cause a flare in symptoms. As intravesical therapy continues, however, this problem usually settles down. There exists a small percentage of patients who just can't tolerate any urethral manipulation whatsoever. This can sometimes be managed by dealing with contributing problems such as vaginal irritations or pelvic floor dysfunction (see chapter 4, Medical Conditions Associated with Interstitial Cystitis).

In rare instances, this urethral pain precludes the use of intravesical therapy.

When Should Intravesical Therapy Be Used?

Should intravesical therapy be used as initial treatment or should it be used only when other therapies fail? There is no good answer to this question. The choice is really up to the clinician's experience and comfort level with the various treatment strategies *and* the patient's preference.

Reasons to Use Intravesical Therapy Initially

* It has few systemic side effects such as fatigue, stomach upset, etc.

* Once the therapy is completed and patients are feeling better, they often can just continue to be observed knowing that they might need to start therapy again if symptoms recur.

* Many patients and clinicians like the concept of a direct approach to the bladder rather than the indirect approach of oral agents.

Reasons to Use Intravesical Therapy as "Second-Line Management"

* It is easier for most patients to take a pill than to come to the doctor's office every week for six to eight consecutive weeks. This can be pretty tough on a work schedule.

* Most patients don't want to even think about getting catheterized unless absolutely necessary.

* Most intravesical therapy is associated with an initial worsening in patient symptoms.

* If the intravesical therapy doesn't work, it means that the patient has devoted a lot of time and emotional energy without reaping any rewards. If oral therapy isn't working, medications can just be stopped and a new one started.

As a general principle, we reserve intravesical therapy for patients in whom less invasive modes of care have failed. However, it is important to understand that the final decision is made during a discussion between clinician and patient. Now, let's discuss the specific agents that are used.

Dimethylsulfoxide (DMSO) RIMSO-50®

Dimethylsulfoxide (DMSO) has been used in the routine management of the IC patient since the 1960s when Stewart, Persky, and Kiser demonstrated the medication's efficacy at reducing IC symptoms (1968). Interestingly, the first use of DMSO entailed rubbing it onto the lower abdomen. It was hoped that the medication would be absorbed and penetrate to the bladder, thereby alleviating symptoms. This didn't work too well, but significant symptom improvement was achieved in the majority of patients who had the DMSO instilled directly into their bladders. Since that time, other investigators have substantiated the efficacy of DMSO in the treatment of IC. For example, Perez-Marrero, Emerson, and Feltis (1988) found that 53 percent of patients had subjective improvement from DMSO therapy. Fowler (1981) also showed that over 80 percent of IC patients improved on this therapy. These studies and others ultimately led to FDA approval for DMSO in the management of interstitial cystitis. Here's a list of some properties of DMSO that make it useful for therapy:

* **Anti-inflammation.** DMSO has anti-inflammatory properties and is also classified as an antioxidant (antioxidants seem to be helpful in cancer prevention). It also causes the release of histamine (a chemical that can stimulate inflammation) from mast cells in the bladder wall. This sounds as if it should cause more inflammation and, indeed, it probably does during the initial treatments; but when all of the

histamine is released, patients may experience improvement in their symptoms.

* **Analgesic effect.** DMSO can deplete substance P from nerves. Substance P is a chemical found in high concentrations in the urine of IC patients. It transmits pain information from nerve to nerve and also stimulates inflammation, a process called neurogenic inflammation (see chapter 3, What Causes Interstitial Cystitis). When substance P is removed, patients may have a reduction in pain. Like its effect on histamine, DMSO may cause an initial increase in substance P, hence it may cause an initial worsening of symptoms. When substance P has been depleted from the nerves, IC symptoms would be expected to decrease.

* **Muscle relaxation.** Spasm of the pelvic muscles (and sometimes of the muscles of the bladder wall) occurs very often in the IC patient. In fact, in many instances, this problem accounts for some of the worst symptoms of urinary urgency, frequency, and pelvic pain. DMSO may be of benefit because it also works as a muscle relaxant.

* **Collagen breakdown.** Collagen is the most abundant protein in our bodies, mainly found in our connective tissues (tendons, joints, and ligaments). It is also important in the process of healing and scar formation. Patients who have the "classical" form of IC may have a large amount of fibrosis (scarring) of the bladder wall. This scarring can decrease the amount of urine that the bladder can hold. DMSO has the ability to break down collagen and hence may be useful at increasing the bladder capacity of some IC patients.

* **Excellent deep penetration into tissues.** DMSO is an excellent solvent that crosses cell membranes with great ease. This means that by placing DMSO in some area of the body, it will rapidly penetrate to deeper layers. That's important when dealing with the IC bladder because we need a medication that can reach the deeper layers, particularly those areas that are rich in nerve fibers and where inflammation might be present. A downside of this property is that DMSO also gets into the bloodstream pretty quickly. Some of the medication is then excreted through your breath. This causes a garlic-like odor that can last for a few hours (in some cases up to twenty-four hours).

* **"Carries" other medications.** As mentioned above, DMSO is an excellent solvent. When other medications are mixed

with it, those medications will often be absorbed to the deeper layers of the bladder along with the DMSO. You'll see how useful this is when the "DMSO cocktail" is discussed.

When DMSO is administered into the bladder, a 50 percent solution is used, called Rimso-50®. Instillations are usually given once per week for six to eight weeks. Some clinicians prefer to instill the agent on an every other week basis. After this period of time, clinicians differ in their approach to further intravesical therapy; however, most suggest some form of "maintenance" dose. For example, assuming that the patient has had a favorable response to therapy, our practice has been to perform another instillation two weeks after the initial six to eight treatments. If the patient continues to do well, the next dose is given three to four weeks later. Overall, the duration between treatments increases until the medication is finally discontinued. There are no hard and fast rules here.

There are some patients whose symptoms rapidly recur with the cessation of DMSO therapy. In those instances, extra treatments are given.

The "DMSO Cocktail"

DMSO has the unique ability to carry other medications along when it is absorbed into tissues. Clinicians have capitalized upon this property by adding other medications to the bladder while instilling the DMSO. This multiagent therapy, also known as the "DMSO cocktail" seems to improve the symptoms in patients who initially failed therapy with DMSO alone (Ghoniem, McBride, Sood, and Lewis 1993). The other medications that are instilled along with the DMSO often include the following:

* **Heparin sulfate.** This is one of the chemicals normally found on the bladder surface. Heparin is actually an anticoagulant (a "blood thinner," meaning that it makes it more difficult for your body to form clots, but also it makes bleeding easier) but when found in the bladder, it seems to serve a protective role on the bladder's surface. When instilled into the bladder, heparin is not absorbed into the body and therefore doesn't have any effect on your ability to bleed. By adding the heparin sulfate to the solution, it is believed that the medication augments the bladder's normal protective surface. Additionally, heparin has anti-inflammatory properties and, like DMSO, it inhibits scar formation.

* **Steroids.** As mentioned in chapter 5's review of oral agents used to treat IC, steroids are potent anti-inflammatory medications. Steroids are often taken orally for diseases associated with inflammation such as rheumatoid arthritis and asthma. They are also used as creams to treat many skin diseases associated with inflammation. Adding a steroid into the DMSO cocktail is like applying creams for skin diseases since the medication is applied directly to the site of the problem. Unlike oral therapy, the steroid is not absorbed throughout the body on a constant basis in high concentrations. The DMSO in the solution presumably carries the steroid to the deeper layers of the bladder wall and, hopefully, decreases any inflammation that might be present.

* **Sodium bicarbonate.** DMSO is a moderately caustic chemical that can irritate the bladder and cause even more bladder symptoms when initially administered. Adding sodium bicarbonate seems to decrease these difficulties.

* **Antibiotics.** Not all clinicians add an antibiotic to the "cocktail." They believe that the chance of acquiring a bladder infection from an instillation is very low and, indeed, it is. We started adding an antibiotic to the DSMO solution when two patients developed an infection midway during their treatment cycles. Both patients were doing very well but the infection caused a flare in symptoms and set the therapy back a few weeks. Needless to say, the patients were disappointed. An antibiotic can be added directly to the solution or can be given as a tablet after the instillation is administered.

What to Expect from DMSO Therapy or a DMSO "Cocktail"

Expect a worsening of symptoms for the first one to three instillations. As discussed above, DMSO is relatively irritating to the bladder surface. Patients often feel worse before they feel better. If you feel great the first time—terrific! If the medication is going to work, we usually see improvement before or at the time of the fourth instillation. Our general policy has been to abort this therapy at this time if no improvement has occurred. Again, these medical strategies vary from clinician to clinician. If pain with DMSO instillation is a problem, it may be a good idea to take a medication for pain prior to your office visit. Taking Pyridium® (see chapter 5, Oral Medications) the day before your office visit may be helpful. On rare occasions, a patient might benefit from taking a narcotic prior to an instillation.

In these instances, you should have someone available to drive you to and from your office visit.

You may not be able to hold the medication(s) in your bladder for a great deal of time. Your clinician will probably ask you to try to hold the medication for about twenty minutes (although the holding times may vary). Don't be disappointed if you can't hold the medication for more than a few minutes. As the therapy progresses, the vast majority of patients will be able to hold the medication for progressively longer periods of time. We've seen patients who, at first, could only hold the medication for one to two minutes. These same patients ended up being able to hold for the full twenty minutes and beyond.

If you feel that your bladder is becoming too full during the instillation, tell your doctor. The total volume of fluid instilled is usually 50–60 cc. This volume might simply be too much for your bladder to hold. Your doctor can adjust for this problem by instilling less volume.

Expect to have bad breath after each treatment. A small amount of DMSO is excreted through the lungs, which gives you a garlic odor on your breath. Interestingly, many patients don't detect the odor, but be assured—those around you do! Keep some mints around. The odor usually lasts two to four hours but it may last as long as twenty-four.

Side Effects of DMSO

DMSO has relatively few side effects apart from causing an initial increase in bladder inflammation. It appears that when used for extended periods of time, there is an increased potential for cataract formation. This information is based solely upon animal studies where very high doses of DMSO were administered. This problem has not been seen in humans. Nevertheless, patients who receive chronic DMSO therapy are advised to undergo periodic eye examinations. Animal studies also suggest that DMSO may cause birth defects. It should, therefore, not be administered during pregnancy.

Heparin Sulfate Instillations

Heparin sulfate as a single agent can be instilled directly into the bladder. This seems to be helpful when the instillations are performed very frequently (three times per week). C. L. Parsons, who popularized this therapy, suggests that patients should have treatments *each day* (Parsons, Housely, Schmidt, and Lebow 1993). When patients have a favorable response (which may take eight to twelve weeks), the frequency of instillations is slowly tapered down. Parsons evaluated forty-eight patients and noted that 56 percent responded favorably to this therapy after twelve weeks. The usual dose of instilled heparin was 10,000 IU mixed in 10 cc sterile water. Symptoms were observed to return within weeks to months of stopping the instillations. This therapy is probably most useful for patients who can't tolerate the DMSO solution due to significant associated symptom flares. Instillations are performed so frequently that patients really need to learn the technique of self-catheterization; otherwise they'll feel as though they are living in the doctor's office.

Heparin Sulfate Injections

Heparin sulfate also has been administered in its injectable form to treat IC. The heparin is usually injected just under the skin (called a *subcutaneous* injection). Studies from Scandinavia have found this therapy useful to decrease the symptoms of IC. All studies have had small numbers of patients (Lose, Jesperson, Frandsen, Hojensgard, et al. 1985; Jesperson and Astrup 1985).

The downside of this approach is that heparin is an anticoagulant. When administered as an injection, much more of this medication gets into the bloodstream than when it is instilled into the bladder (actually, virtually no heparin works its way into the bloodstream when instilled into the bladder). Patients might therefore notice that they bruise easier, and their gums might bleed when they brush their teeth. When these problems occur, the heparin dose should be lowered or the drug discontinued. Additionally, long-term use of heparin is associated with osteoporosis. The frequency of heparin injections used clinically varies from several times per week to several times per day. No studies have been conducted to determine the optimal dosing schedule.

The Anesthetic Cocktail

The anesthetic cocktail may be simply a mixture of a short-acting anesthetic such as lidocaine (Xylocaine®) and a long-acting anesthetic like bupivacaine (Marcaine®). Some clinicians also add many of the agents used in the DMSO cocktail such as heparin sulfate, a steroid, and an antibiotic (but not the DMSO).

The best part about receiving this solution is that pain relief, if it is going to occur, takes place within minutes. Based upon the duration of action of the anesthetic agents, one might imagine that the symptom relief achieved would last only about three to four hours.

Interestingly, many patients have a reduction in symptoms that lasts for several days to a week or more.

The anesthetic cocktail is useful in two instances. First, instillation of the anesthetic medications can help determine the source of pelvic pain. When a patient has significant symptom relief from the solution, it implies very strongly that the origin of the pain is indeed the bladder. Second, the anesthetic cocktail can be used for therapy just as with DMSO treatments. The downside here is that in some instances the solution may need to be administered more than once per week. The anesthetic cocktail has been particularly helpful as emergency therapy for those patients who are experiencing a flare in their symptoms.

One final word of caution about the anesthetic cocktail—sometimes the instillation can work too well. We once had a patient who had a very severe case of IC, associated with a very tiny bladder and Hunner's ulcers (red patches on the bladder surface that correspond to intense inflammation). She typically voided every ten minutes both day and night and was experiencing worsening pelvic pain. We instilled the anesthetic cocktail and within minutes she felt terrific. We asked her to hold the medication in for twenty minutes (if she could even do that) and then to urinate the solution out.

Well, the patient went home from the office and felt so great that apparently she decided to hold the medications in her bladder for over two hours! She called us up concerned about the passage of large blood clots in her urine. The reason this patient started to bleed was that she held the solution in her bladder far too long. Her bladder was very small. By holding off urinating for so long, she actually overstretched her bladder and caused some bleeding. She did just fine by drinking lots of fluid. This anecdote points out how useful this instillation can be *and* that there are potential problems.

Iontophoresis: An Interesting Way to Enhance the Effect of Intravesical Anesthetics

Iontophoresis, also called *electromotive drug administration* (EMDA), usually involves employing a small amount of electricity to enhance the penetration of a drug. In the case of the IC bladder, a medication such as an anesthetic is instilled into the bladder through a special catheter that contains an electrode (see figure 9). Small patches are then placed on the skin and a small electrical current is then established from the catheter to those patches. The electrical current drags the medication (in most cases an anesthetic) along into the deeper layers of the bladder, bypassing the bladder's normal protective lining.

Using this technique, certain surgical procedures for the bladder can be performed without using conventional anesthesia (such as a general or spinal anesthesia). Likewise, hydrodistention of the bladder can be performed on IC patients. One study performed EMDA on twenty-five patients with different types of "noninfectious cystitis" of whom sixteen were IC patients. A total of sixty-five treatments were performed. The group reported a 60 percent complete remission (complete absence of symptoms) rate and a 12 percent partial remission rate that lasted an average of 6.6 months. The bladder capacity was increased by 173 percent (Riedl, Knoll, Plas, and Pflòger 1998). The investigators noted that a temporary worsening of urinary symptoms was common. All patients had redness at the site where the patch electrodes were placed. A few patients had a second-degree burn (associated with skin blistering) at that site.

Iontophoresis appears to be an up-and-coming technique that has definite potential for the treatment of IC. Hopefully, it is a technology that will soon be available as standard therapy in the United States.

BCG (Bacillus Calmette-Guérin)

Bacillus Calmette-Guérin (BCG) is routinely used in the management of bladder cancer. BCG is not chemotherapy for the bladder. Rather, it is the tuberculosis bacterium that is treated in such a fashion as to dramatically decrease its ability to cause tuberculosis. It is instilled into the bladder and can kill bladder cancer cells and/or prevent their recurrence. Recent studies by Peters, Diokno, Steinert, and Gonzales (1998) at Beaumont Hospital, Detroit, suggest that this therapy can be useful to many IC patients. In 1998 they reported that about 60 percent of IC patients had a favorable response to BCG as opposed to a 27 percent favorable response rate in those patients receiving a placebo (sterile saline). Daily voids decreased by 31 percent; pelvic pain decreased by 81 percent; evening voids decreased by 54 percent; urgency decreased by 71 percent. Of the nine patients who had a favorable response to the BCG, eight of the nine (89 percent) had continued symptom improvement for an average follow-up time of twenty-seven months. *All pretty spectacular results!* Of those patients who had no response to the BCG, no worsening of symptoms was seen.

The biggest concern about intravesical BCG is its ability to cause tuberculosis throughout the body (called "BCG sepsis"). This problem rarely has been seen in patients receiving this form of

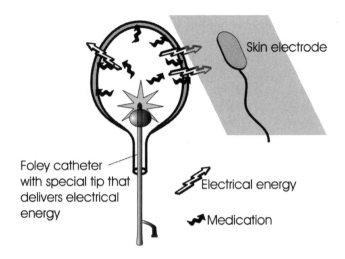

Figure 9. Iontophoresis. A low voltage electrical current runs between the bladder catheter and the skin electrode. Medications are carried along with the electrical current into the deeper layers of the bladder wall.

therapy for bladder cancer, and has never been seen in an IC patient. BCG sepsis can be life-threatening or even lethal and occurs due to the BCG getting into the bloodstream. Most practitioners do not use BCG in the early management of the IC patient because of these potential risks and the fact that the encouraging results seen with BCG therapy have not yet been verified in large numbers of patients at other institutions (these studies are now underway).

Capsaicin

Did you ever notice what happens when you bite into a hot pepper? At first you feel as though you'd like to have a tongue transplant. After a few minutes, you may notice that your tongue has lost a lot of its sensitivity. That effect is caused by capsaicin. Capsaicin is the pungent component of the hot pepper. When capsaicin comes into contact with your tongue or is instilled into your bladder, substance P is released (remember, substance P carries pain messages through the nerves and stimulates inflammation). When the substance P has all been released, you're left (hopefully) with less pain. If the pain-carrying nerves are repeatedly exposed to capsaicin, these nerves might stop functioning altogether.

Capsaicin may also decrease sensitivity by its action as a "counterirritant." A counterirritant is a substance that causes an irritation but by doing so it decreases other types of coexisting pain. In a very general sense, this is akin to curing a headache by hitting your thumb with a hammer.

Capsaicin therapy was first popularized in Ferrara, Italy. In 1989, Maggi, Barbanti, Santicioli, Beneforte, et al. instilled a dilute capsaicin solution into the bladders of five patients suffering from bladder "hypersensitivity." Four of the five patients had complete disappearance of their symptoms. The fifth patient had a "marked" attenuation of symptoms (including pain, urinary frequency, urgency, etc.). Symptom relief lasted four to sixteen days.

In 1998, Lazzeri, Benforte, Turini, Spinelli, et al. investigated the use of intravesical capsaicin in the management of severe bladder pain. They evaluated thirty-six patients who either received saline or a dilute capsaicin solution (patients didn't know which medication that they were to receive) two times per week for one month. Patients were evaluated at the end of one month and again at six months. Significant decreases in urinary daytime and nighttime frequency were seen but there was no evidence of any significant change in urinary urgency or bladder pain. Lazzeri's group was concerned that the unimpressive results were due to a capsaicin dose that was too low. In 1997, Cruz, Guimarâes, Silva, Edite Rio, et al. used a much higher dose (1 mM). They instilled this solution into the bladders of sixteen patients, three of whom had "bladder hypersensitivity." All three of these patients faired well on this therapy. Two felt "much better"; one felt slightly better. All patients had impressive increases in their bladder capacities. The problem with this study is certainly its small number of patients. More importantly, the dose of capsaicin was so high that patients had a difficult time with severe bladder burning during the instillations. When using lower capsaicin concentrations, an anesthetic is instilled into the bladder and held for fifteen to thirty minutes prior to instilling the capsaicin. Unfortunately, when the dose of capsaicin is very high, not even this anesthetic can relieve associated pain.

Flood, Shupp-Byrne, Rivas, McCue, et al. in 1997 evaluated ten patients undergoing therapy with higher doses of capsaicin (2 mM). Treatments started at low doses on a twice per week basis. As the treatments continued (for a total of four weeks) the doses of capsaicin instilled in to the bladder progressively increased. At the end of the study, five of the ten patients noted a greater or equal to 50 percent improvement in pain. Additionally, voiding diaries of these patients demonstrated a greater or equal to 50 percent improvement in urinary frequency.

Our experience (seven patients) and anecdotal reports of others demonstrated that patients still experienced a moderate amount of "bladder burning," even after the anesthetic was instilled. Patients did not seem to fare much better than with DMSO therapy. Consequently, we have not made routine use of this treatment.

Resiniferatoxin

Resiniferatoxin has a very similar action to capsaicin but it's about 1,000 times more potent. Given what you have just read about capsaicin, you might be wondering how in the world this agent could ever be tolerated in someone's bladder. Actually, it does seem to be well tolerated and doesn't have the associated burning that capsaicin does. Trials are presently underway to determine the role of this medication in the treatment of IC.

Cromolyn Sodium (Gastrocrom®)

Cromolyn sodium is used routinely to treat asthma. It seems to work by preventing the release of inflammation-causing substances, such as histamine, from mast cells. In chapter 3, What Causes Interstitial Cystitis?, we discussed the fact that IC patients tend to have higher levels of histamine and higher numbers of mast cells in their bladder walls. Edwards, Bucknall, and Makin (1986) evaluated nine IC patients with severe symptoms (bladder removal was contemplated in all of these patients). Four percent sodium cromoglycate was instilled into their bladders each day for twelve days. Patients retained the solution for at least one hour during each session. No patient reported any pain when the medication was instilled. Of the nine patients, two had complete resolution of their symptoms. One of these patients remained symptom-free for over two years. Four patients had a partial relief in symptoms, but still required some other medical treatments. The remaining three patients had no symptom relief.

Another study by Kennelly and Konnack (1995), examined the effects of 10 percent cromolyn instilled on a daily basis for one month. Seven IC patients received the cromolyn and nine IC patients received placebo. Of the seven patients who had the true drug instilled, three had greater than a 75 percent improvement in symptoms. Only one of the nine patients receiving placebo showed such an improvement.

Overall, these investigations suggest that intravesical instillation of cromolyn can be helpful in a certain group of IC patients. This intervention appears to be rather "benign," with its major drawback being the very frequent medication instillations required (daily as per the above studies). Larger studies need to be performed to determine the ultimate role of this therapy in standard management.

Hyaluronic Acid (Cystistat®)

Hyaluronic acid is found in high quantities in bladder surface mucin, the protective chemical lining of the bladder. Like heparin sulfate, hyaluronic acid has many other qualities that make it potentially useful in the treatment of interstitial cystitis. For example, it seems to decrease scar formation; it promotes connective tissue healing; it has anti-inflammatory qualities, and it is an antioxidant. In 1997, Morales, Emerson, and Nickel conducted a trial of intravesical hyaluronic acid in IC patients who had failed to improve with many other therapies. Twenty-five patients received 40 mg of hyaluronic acid into their bladders each week for four weeks; then on a monthly basis. After four weeks of therapy, 56 percent of patients had either a complete or partial response. This percentage increased to 71 percent by the twelfth week of therapy. A decrease in the efficacy of the medication was seen after that point in time.

Another study by Porru, Campus, Tudino, Valdes, et al. (1997) evaluated ten patients undergoing intravesical hyaluronic acid therapy. Those patients received weekly instillations of 40 mg hyaluronic acid for six weeks. They noted that 30 percent of patients improved and this improvement continued during an observation period of six months. The medication in both investigations was well tolerated.

In summary, hyaluronic acid therapy appears to be effective in some IC patients. Long-term studies with more patients are needed to better assess the efficacy of this treatment and to determine the characteristics of those patients who are more likely to have a favorable response. Cystistat is available in Canada but not in the United States. It can be obtained by mail order (Bioniche, Montreal, Quebec, Canada). Another similar therapy being used in Canada is the intravesical instillation of chondroitin sulfate (Stellar International, Inc. London, Ontario). The medication is Uracyst-S (0.2% chondroitin sulfate). Clinical trials are underway to determine its efficacy at reducing IC symptoms.

Silver Nitrate (and Argyrol®)

Silver nitrate was the first intravesical therapy used to treat the IC patient. The solution is very caustic and when given in high concentrations can cause bladder scarring. In fact it's so caustic that a test called a cystogram must be performed prior to the instillation. A cystogram is an x-ray taken while the bladder is full of an x-ray contrast solution. The test is performed to ensure that no fluid can move up the ureters and then up to the kidneys, a condition known as *reflux*. (In the normal situation this cannot occur. Urine flows only from the kidneys to the bladder.) If the contrast solution is seen in either or both ureters, the ureters must be blocked off to ensure that the silver nitrate doesn't travel up there. Silver nitrate in the ureter easily can lead to scaring and to ultimate blockage of the ureter from the scar. The cystogram is usually performed while the patient is asleep, at the time of the silver nitrate instillation.

Some investigators have advocated performing the instillations in the office after anesthetizing the bladder surface. The concentration of silver nitrate used for instillation varies from 1:5000 (1 part silver nitrate to 5000 parts water) to 1:50. The number of treatments varies from one to multiple, depending upon the clinician's interpretation of the literature. Symptomatic improvement has been noted ranging from 50–93 percent. Recurrence of symptoms necessitating the use of other therapies is common.

Why caustic chemicals like silver nitrate or Clorpactin (see text below) improve the symptoms of IC is unknown. Some possibilities include the following:

* They cause a great deal of damage to the bladder surface. When the bladder repairs itself, the new lining functions better. Recent studies in our laboratory have demonstrated significant increases in GP51 content in the urine of IC patients *after* the bladder surface has been damaged. GP51 is a chemical that is found on the bladder surface (part of bladder surface mucin) and probably has some role in protecting the underlying bladder cells.

* These medications destroy the nerves of the bladder.

* Much like capsaicin, these medications cause the release of substance P. This ultimately leads to a decrease in inflammation and in the transmission of pain.

The concern about using these medications is their tendency to cause scarring and even to stimulate the growth of *more* nerves at a later date. These medications are therefore not generally used as first-line therapy.

Argyrol ("mild silver protein solution") has been used by some practitioners as intravesical therapy for interstitial cystitis. This medication is not at all related to silver nitrate. It is much less caustic and therefore can be administered without anesthesia. Argyrol was originally marketed as a topical antiseptic and was used by ophthalmologists to treat the eye prior to surgery. The medication was ultimately found to be poor at killing germs and is used infrequently today. Although anecdotal reports of Argyrol's efficacy in the treatment of IC exist, no clinical studies are available for review.

Sodium Oxychlorosene
(Clorpactin WCS-90®)

Clorpactin® was originally used to treat severe bladder infections in the days prior to antibiotics. For example, tuberculosis of the urinary tract is a serious illness that can cause many of the same symptoms as interstitial cystitis. In the days when tuberculosis was much more prevalent, urine cultures were always tested for it. Clorpactin kills most microorganisms on contact. This agent is chemically similar to dilute chlorine bleach. Although most people think that chlorine bleach is highly poisonous, it's actually relatively nontoxic (although we wouldn't try testing this out). Clorpactin was originally instilled into the bladders of IC patients on the premise that it would kill an undiagnosed microorganism (Wishard, Nourse, and Mertz 1957) but today we feel that other mechanisms account for its ability to decrease the symptoms of interstitial cystitis.

Like the use of silver nitrate, strategies to instill the medication vary considerably. The concentration of Clorpactin used has usually ranged from a 0.2 percent solution to a 0.4 percent solution. In a study by Messing and Stamey (1978), thirty-eight patients were treated with multiple treatments using a 0.4 percent solution of Clorpactin. They reported that 72 percent of patients had at least a six-month improvement in symptoms.

La Rock and Sant (1997) report that long-term remission is seen in about 30 percent of patients. Their protocol for Clorpactin therapy uses a 0.4 percent solution. This is instilled while the patient receives general anesthesia (the patient is asleep). The medication remains in the bladder for about four to seven minutes. It's then drained from the bladder. This process is repeated about three to four times for a total "contact" time of fifteen to twenty minutes. Patients typically complain of urinary urgency, frequency, burning, and pelvic pain after the procedure.

A catheter is left in place for one to two days post-operatively. The catheter is connected to a small drainage bag that is attached to the leg (also known as a "leg bag"). The catheter is placed on a temporary basis until the bladder inflammation settles down. In the meantime, patients are given pain medications to decrease their level of discomfort. In La Rock and Sant's hands, 50–60 percent of patients had a "meaningful" symptomatic improvement from this therapy.

Additionally, Dr. Sant's experience in treating over eighty IC patients with multiple courses of Clorpactin therapy (up to eight to ten times) demonstrated no ill effects to the bladder (for example, no reduction in bladder capacity, no abnormalities of the bladder surface).

The disadvantage of Clorpactin is that, like silver nitrate, it usually needs to be instilled under anesthesia. The ureters also need to be blocked off temporarily if ureteral reflux is present. That means that the same x-ray testing must be performed as for silver nitrate. Clorpactin is probably most useful for the patient who has failed other less aggressive forms of management such as DMSO therapy.

The Usefulness of Self-Catheterization

As you have probably surmised by now, intravesical therapy involves a lot of work. Many IC patients live considerable distances from their clinicians. Simply stated, it's just a big pain in the neck to get to the office so often (especially with those ridiculous waiting times!). When bladder instillations are performed on a chronic basis, it's often a good idea to learn how to administer the medication yourself. Of course, not all patients are that keen on learning this technique. Additionally, patients who have a great deal of associated urethral pain are probably not good candidates for self-catheterization.

On the other hand, a motivated patient without urethral pain usually does just fine with a few simple lessons. Apart from its usefulness for instilling medicines into the bladder, learning self-catheterization also can be tremendously helpful to the patient who occasionally can't urinate at all (also known as urinary retention). When urinary retention occurs, patients usually need to go to the closest emergency room to have a catheter placed. If you know how to place the catheter yourself, and you have the catheter at home, you can deal with the problem within a few minutes. Note that the technique of self-catheterization is best taught by experienced medical personnel.

Chapter 7

The Male with Interstitial Cystitis

Unfortunately, the male IC patient often has more difficulty receiving a diagnosis and ultimate treatment than the female IC patient. The reason for this is simple. Interstitial cystitis is more commonly seen in females. In fact, many clinicians think of IC as a "female illness," and, therefore, overlook the possibility of IC in their male patients. Another difficulty is that men have other common problems that can cause symptoms identical to interstitial cystitis. This can lead to confusion in establishing a correct diagnosis. In fact, in a 1969 review of 123 male IC patients, Hanash and Pool noted that 55 percent of these men had had at least one scraping of their prostate glands (a procedure called a transurethral resection of the prostate, or TURP). The patients had undergone these surgical procedures because their symptoms had been attributed to prostatic enlargement. However, the men in this study had shown no significant improvement in their symptoms after prostate scraping. That's when the light bulbs went on—maybe something else was going on.

To make the diagnosis of IC in the male patient even more problematic, it's possible to have two problems at the same time, such as IC and a prostate that's obstructing the flow of urine. For these reasons a very careful evaluation of the male must be performed before reaching a diagnosis of interstitial cystitis. Of course, the first step is to include IC in the list of possibilities. In the study by Hanash and Pool, interstitial cystitis had been suspected in only 17 percent of the patients when they were first seen.

Fortunately, over the past several years, many clinicians have developed a heightened awareness of IC in the male. We're now seeing more and more patients who have been treated for problems such as "prostatitis" or prostate enlargement without success. Many of these patients are ultimately diagnosed with IC after being medically evaluated.

Let's now run through some medical problems commonly seen in men that can mimic interstitial cystitis. These can be broadly divided into diseases of the prostate, bladder, seminal vesicles, and pelvic floor muscles.

The Prostate Gland

The prostate gland sits under the bladder and weighs about 25–30 grams in the adult male. It has many functions, some of which include the following:

1. Creation of about 15 percent of the semen volume.

2. Shortly after ejaculation, the semen becomes rather "thick" in consistency. Enzymes secreted by the prostate liquefy the semen again.

3. The prostate contains the highest levels of zinc in the body. "Free" zinc is the zinc ion that is not "bound" to other chemicals; it also has antibacterial properties. It's believed that the prostate may, therefore, help in the prevention of urinary tract infections.

4. Muscle tissue in and around the prostate appears to serve a role in the maintenance of urinary continence (the ability to hold urine in your bladder without leakage).

Prostate Disorders That Mimic Interstitial Cystitis

Almost any medical illness related to the prostate can give rise to symptoms indistinguishable from interstitial cystitis. The problems discussed below are all commonly seen in urological practice. Interstitial cystitis is usually suspected when there is limited or no symptom improvement with traditional therapy.

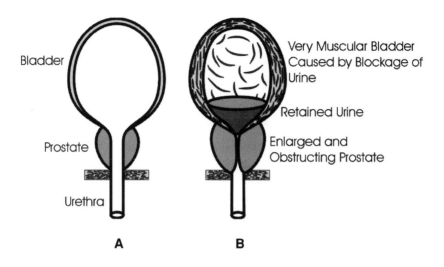

Bladder

Prostate

Urethra

Very Muscular Bladder Caused by Blockage of Urine

Retained Urine

Enlarged and Obstructing Prostate

A   **B**

Figure 10. A. The normal bladder, urethra, and prostate. B. Prostate growth causing blockage of urine flow through the urethra. The bladder needs to contract harder in order to push urine out. In some instances, the bladder just can't push hard enough to completely empty—some urine remains in the bladder after voiding.

Prostate Enlargement (Also called Benign Prostatic Hyperplasia, or BPH)

Enlargement of the prostate occurs in all men with normally functioning testicles. A derivative of the testosterone produced in the testicles called dihydrotestosterone stimulates prostatic growth. Benign prostatic hyperplasia (BPH) appears to begin rather early in life, even in twenty- and thirty-year-olds and continues over the ensuing years. Growth of the prostate gland doesn't generally cause symptoms until the fifties (there are, however, plenty of exceptions). At that time, the enlarging prostate can slowly begin to block the passage of urine through the urethra (see figure 10). It's important to note here that some men have much more prostate growth than other men. Also, keep in mind that just because the prostate grows in size doesn't mean that the urethra is always blocked off. You can have a very large prostate associated with no voiding problems at all. Conversely, a small prostate easily can cause significant obstruction to urine flow if the growth occurs "inward" into the urethra.

When problems related to BPH occur, symptoms are usually of two varieties: obstructive and/or irritative.

Obstructive voiding symptoms. These are symptoms that relate directly to the blockage of urine flow. Examples of these symptoms include the following:

1. Difficulty initiating the urine stream—also called "urinary hesitancy." This is often more of a problem first thing in the morning.

2. Poor force of the urine stream.

3. Sensation of incomplete emptying.

4. The need to strain when urinating.

5. A lot of urine dribbling after the initial urine stream (also called "post-void dribbling").

It is interesting that many of these symptoms sound like the symptoms of patients with pelvic floor dysfunction, a problem commonly associated with IC (see chapter 4, Medical Conditions Associated with Interstitial Cystitis).

Irritative voiding symptoms. When the flow of urine is obstructed by the prostate, the bladder often compensates by pushing with more force. In many instances, this compensation keeps the urine flow pretty strong, and you may not even sense that a problem exists. On the other hand, that good urine flow rate often comes at a price. As the blockage continues, the bladder muscle (remember, the bladder is comprised mostly of muscle) starts to thicken and becomes more powerful. If the clinician performs cystoscopy, he/she might see large bands of muscle poking through the normally smooth bladder surface, called *bladder trabeculation*. At this point, the bladder frequently starts to contract at inappropriate times. Terms that describe this bladder behavior include "bladder instability" or the "overactive bladder." Examples of the irritative voiding symptoms that result include the following:

1. Sudden urges to void ("urinary urgency").

2. Urinary frequency—typically small volumes are voided each time.

3. Going to the bathroom several times per night, typically small volumes.

4. Leakage of urine because of the inability to hold back the sudden urge to urinate.

Besides the urinary leakage (which occurs rarely), these irritative voiding symptoms sound just like those produced by interstitial cystitis. You can see why many clinicians, when hearing these types of complaints, might begin an evaluation for prostatic blockage, rather than for interstitial cystitis. That's perfectly good medical care, especially for the following reasons:

1. BPH is far more common than interstitial cystitis.

2. BPH can coexist with interstitial cystitis.

3. Ultimately, other difficulties can occur as a result of BPH, such as the following:

   * **Acute urinary retention**. In this situation, the patient suddenly can't urinate at all or can produce only drops. This is usually associated with lower abdominal pain. The lower abdomen hurts when examined (that's because the bladder is filled to its maximum capacity with urine) and a urethral catheter is usually placed to empty the bladder and make the patient comfortable again. The reason that this condition develops is not always apparent; however, urinary tract infections, urological instrumentation (such as an office cystoscopy), or the use of cold remedies can sometimes be the culprits. (Often cold medications have ingredients that can weaken the bladder's ability to contract or tighten the neck of the bladder—both conditions leading to a worsening of the urine flow. So *watch out!* Be sure to read the cold remedy label. These medications are reviewed later in this chapter under "Differences Between Men and Women in the Treatment of IC.")

   * **Loss of bladder function/chronic urinary retention**. In the face of chronic obstruction, sometimes the bladder just can't squeeze hard enough. It starts to loose it's ability to contract well. The consequence is a bladder that doesn't empty to completion. Rarely, this can result in a bladder that loses all of its ability to contract. In some cases, the bladder can be "rehabilitated" to contract again. Unfortunately, in other cases, the bladder's function cannot be reclaimed. This can lead to the following problems:

   * **Urinary tract infections**. When the bladder doesn't empty well, any bacteria that gain access to it have a better chance of multiplying and causing an infection.

   * **Kidney damage**. In rare instances, chronic urinary retention can be of such magnitude that urine actually backs

up to the kidneys. Under normal circumstances, urine travels only in one direction—from the kidneys, down to the bladder. But when high pressures build up in the bladder for long periods of time, the valve that keeps the urine flowing in one direction fails. This allows the kidney to be exposed to high pressures of urine, which may ultimately lead to kidney failure. Fortunately, this is a rare event.

 * **Bladder stones.** Bladder stones form when the bladder doesn't empty well and the urine becomes concentrated. This is a perfect situation for chemicals like calcium oxalate to come out of solution and form microscopic crystals, much like "rock candy" made from a concentrated sugar solution. The crystals can become larger with time and ultimately form large stones within the bladder. The bladder stones, themselves, can cause irritative voiding symptoms.

Treatment for the Prostate That Is Obstructing the Flow of Urine

If your clinician thinks that prostatic obstruction is present, several options of care are available such as:

1. **Observation.** About 10–15 percent of patients actually have improvement in their symptoms over time.

2. **Medications.** The most common medication used to improve the symptoms of BPH are the alpha-blockers (see chapter 5, Oral Medications). These medications usually will improve the obstructive symptoms quickly, but it may take a lot longer to see the effect on the irritative voiding symptoms. Other medications are available to decrease the size of the prostate such as Proscar® (finasteride). This latter medication isn't used quite as much these days for BPH management because the improvement in the urine stream can take three to six months to take place. Herbal remedies such as Saw palmetto (*Serenoa repens*) and *Pygeum africanum* appear to work in a similar fashion.

3. **Surgery.** This treatment option is usually not considered unless medical therapy fails. A full review of the surgical options for BPH is beyond the scope of this text, but here's a listing of some procedures that are available. They range

from the least to the most invasive. Overall, the most invasive procedures tend to yield the "best results" (best relief of symptoms for the longest period of time) and vise versa.

* **Transurethral microwave thermotherapy.** An outpatient procedure where a catheter is placed into the urethra. There is a microwave coil placed within the catheter. The coil discharges microwave energy into the prostate, causing many of the cells within the prostate to die. When this occurs, there is less compression of the urethra by the prostate, and urine flow increases.

* **Transurethral needle ablation (TUNA).** This outpatient procedure works along the same principle as microwave thermotherapy. In this instance, small needles are inserted into the prostate and low-level radio frequency energy is delivered.

* **Laser coagulation of the prostate.** As the name implies, laser energy is applied to the prostate through a special cystoscope. The cells die and, as with microwave thermotherapy and TUNA, the urethral passage opens.

* **Transurethral incision of the prostate.** A special cystoscope, called a resectoscope, is used to create one to three incisions at the neck of the bladder and in the prostate. The urethra often "springs open" after these incisions have been made, thus allowing easier passage of urine.

* **Transurethral vaporization of the prostate.** This procedure is similar to the TURP (see below) but uses a special electrode that comes in contact with the prostate. The electrode delivers high energy to the tissue which causes it to vaporize, thus creating an open channel for the flow of urine.

* **Transurethral resection of the prostate (TURP).** This is the "gold standard" procedure to deal with prostatic obstruction. It involves using a resectoscope to "scrape" away obstructing prostatic tissue—much like coring out an apple.

* **Open prostatectomy.** Open surgery to deal with an obstructing prostate usually is performed when the prostate gland is very large, a situation where lesser invasive forms of therapy will be likely to fail. When open prostatectomy is performed, only the central portion of the gland is removed. The outer portion is left in place just as with the TURP.

The patient makes the final choice of therapy after a discussion involving the pros and cons of each.

One symptom that frequently sets the IC patient apart from the typical patient who suffers from BPH is pain. Pelvic pain, specifically related to the male, is usually derived from other diseases of the prostate such as cancer, inflammation, or infection. So, let's now discuss those issues.

Inflammation of the Prostate (Prostatitis)

Prostatitis, like interstitial cystitis, is a medical illness whose diagnosis is sometimes difficult to achieve, and, in many cases, therapy is not all that successful. Its symptoms can be remarkably similar to interstitial cystitis. Prostatitis can be broken down into the following four basic categories:

1. **Acute bacterial prostatitis (recently reclassified as Category I Prostatitis).** This form of prostatitis is always associated with a urinary tract infection. The patient typically has a fever. The prostate is hot and tender when a rectal examination is performed. Due to prostatic swelling, the urine stream can be partially or totally blocked off. Patients with acute prostatitis frequently need to be hospitalized and placed on intravenous antibiotics. This form of prostatitis is never confused with interstitial cystitis.

2. **Chronic bacterial prostatitis (reclassified as Category II Prostatitis).** Category II prostatitis is characterized by a smoldering bacterial infection within the prostate gland, usually associated with periodic urinary tract infections. If the prostate gland is squeezed during a "vigorous" (and not particularly enjoyable) rectal exam (called, perhaps inappropriately, "prostatic massage"), prostatic secretions can be obtained. When cultured, these secretions demonstrate bacteria and other signs of infection. When these patients do not have an overt infection, they may still have signs and symptoms that include the following:

   * Occasional discharge from the urethra

   * Occasional burning when urinating

   * Scrotal/testicular pain

   * Perineal discomfort (area between the anus and scrotum)

* Lower back pain

* Urinary frequency

* Urinary urgency

* Lower abdominal discomfort

* Penile pain

* Pain with ejaculation

Therapy for this form of prostatitis involves long courses of antibiotics, ranging from six weeks to three months. The success of antibiotic therapy (usually with a group of medications called the fluoroquinolones is about 70 to 90 percent. Examples of medications in this group include Noroxin®, Cipro®, Levaquin®, Tequin®, and Floxin®). Unfortunately, relapses of infection are common.

Category II prostatitis is often difficult to eradicate for several reasons including the following:

* Many antibiotics can't penetrate into prostatic tissue well. For example, antibiotics typically used to deal with uncomplicated urinary tract infections such as amoxicillin and Macrodantin® don't penetrate into prostatic tissue at all in this setting. The fluoroquinolones (and a few other classes of antibiotics) have excellent penetration into this tissue but other factors listed below can still make achieving a cure difficult.

* Nickel, Downey, Clark, Ceri, et al. (1995) found that bacteria within the prostate may encase themselves in an antibiotic-resistant substance called a "biofilm." There is some evidence that these bacteria also slow down their metabolism, making them more resistant to the effects of antibiotics.

* Many men normally have calcifications within their prostate glands called *prostatic calculi*. Bacteria can migrate into these calcifications which serve as a barrier against antibiotic penetration.

When many people think of "prostatitis," this is the form of the disease that usually comes to mind. In reality, Category II prostatitis is relatively uncommon, accounting for only about 5 percent of prostatitis patients. By far, the most common form of prostatitis seen by clinicians is MCPPS (male chronic pelvic pain syndrome) Category III, accounting for more than 85 percent of patients with a "prostatitis syndrome."

3. **Male chronic pelvic pain syndrome, Category III.** Patients with this disorder have many of the symptoms seen in Category II prostatitis, but in this instance there is no evidence of infection. This group of patients has been divided into the following two categories:

  * **Nonbacterial prostatitis (reclassified as MCPPS, Category IIIA).** No infection is seen in the prostatic secretions; however, inflammatory cells are present. This finding is strongly suggestive of an inflammatory process within the prostate.

  * **Prostatodynia (reclassified as MCPPS, Category IIIB).** Patients have all the symptoms of a prostatic infection but there's no evidence of any inflammation or infection of the prostate. The symptoms, in most instances, are attributable to spasm of the pelvic floor muscles (see chapter 4, Medical Conditions Associated with Interstitial Cystitis).

4. **Asymptomatic inflammatory prostatitis (now categorized as Category IV Prostatitis).** These patients have no symptoms at all. In this instance, inflammation of the prostate is found incidentally during the evaluation of some other prostatic problem. By far, this form of prostatitis is most commonly diagnosed during the evaluation of prostate cancer. A patient typically has a biopsy of the prostate performed. The biopsy doesn't demonstrate cancer but it does show prostatic inflammation. No therapy is warranted in these instances.

Can Prostatitis and IC be Related Problems?

Let's take a look back at the category termed "Male Chronic Pelvic Pain Syndrome, Type III." Like interstitial cystitis, these problems (both categories IIIA and IIIB) have been a diagnostic and therapeutic dilemma for clinicians. Treatments have ranged from empirical antibiotic therapy to anti-inflammatory medications to physical therapy to microwave therapy of the prostate gland.

In 1987, Messing suggested that some men with MCPPS, Category IIIB (prostatodynia) might actually have interstitial cystitis. Although patients with MCPPS, Category III prostatitis don't usually complain of bladder symptoms (such as pain with bladder filling, urinary urgency or frequency), Siroky, Goldstein, and Krane (1981)

Table 7.1:   Comparison Between MCPPS, Category III and Interstitial Cystitis

Symptoms	IC		MCPPS, Category III
	Urinary urgency, frequency, pelvic pain, pain with sexual intercourse		Pelvic pain, perineal pain, testicular pain, penile pain, pain with intercourse (ejaculation)
Pain with bladder filling	Almost always		45 percent of patients
Urine culture	Negative		Negative
Office cystoscopy findings	No abnormalities		No abnormalities
Pain from pelvic floor muscles	Frequently seen		Frequently seen
Signs of inflammation	Variable		Variable

reproduced the pelvic pain in 45 percent of patients by filling the bladder with fluid (sounds very much like IC, doesn't it?). A basic comparison between these two medical conditions is outlined in the table above.

As you can easily see, many similarities exist between these two problems. Miller, Rothman, Bavendam, and Berger (1995) from the University of Washington–Seattle, took this comparison one step further by performing a bladder hydrodistention on thirty-eight men who had been diagnosed with MCPPS, Category III. Sixty-three percent of these men were found to have moderate to severe glomerulations (small bleeding points on the bladder surface that are frequently seen in IC patients). Most of the men who had these findings suggestive of interstitial cystitis had no significant inflammation of the prostate, putting them into the Category IIIB (prostatodynia) group. What's really interesting about this information is how it compares to our previous work demonstrating that 70 percent of

IC patients have associated pelvic floor dysfunction (the pain of prostatodynia is thought to be caused by spasm of the pelvic floor muscles).

So, what should you take away from all of this information? The important point here is that there are many patients who have been diagnosed with prostatitis (particularly MCPPS, Category IIIB) who have not responded to therapy. A body of evidence is mounting that suggests some of these patients may indeed have interstitial cystitis. If the diagnosis of IC is ultimately made, other forms of therapy become available that may result in good symptom improvement.

Seminal Vesiculitis

The seminal vesicles are structures that connect to the prostate gland and sit behind the bladder. Their function is not completely understood but we do know that they connect with the vas deferens (the tube that brings sperm from the testicles) and create the majority of the liquid portion of the semen. The fluid that the seminal vesicles create is high in the sugar fructose and in prostaglandin E.

Seminal vesiculitis means inflammation of the seminal vesicles. This is a nonspecific term, failing to describe the cause of the inflammation. In most instances, seminal vesiculitis is accompanied by prostatitis. And just as with prostatitis, seminal vesiculitis can be caused by an infection *or* the inflammation might be present without any evidence of infection. Symptoms of seminal vesiculitis can sound much like interstitial cystitis and include the following:

* Urinary frequency

* Poor urine flow

* Pain with or after ejaculation

* Sensation of incomplete bladder emptying

* Blood in the urine or in the semen

* Pain with urination

* Testicular or perineal pain

* Low back pain

Normally, one cannot feel the seminal vesicles upon rectal examination, however, in the presence of seminal vesiculitis, these structures often are easy to feel and are usually pretty tender. Because prostatitis is frequently present at the same time, the prostate might also be tender. An ultrasound evaluation of the prostate and seminal vesicles can be performed to better evaluate this region.

This test usually employs an ultrasound "probe" that's advanced into the rectum with lots of lubricating jelly—hence the term, "transrectal ultrasonography (or TRUS)." The seminal vesicles and prostate can be visualized easily by this method because these structures are on the other side of the rectal wall. When seminal vesiculitis is present, TRUS often demonstrates the seminal vesicles to be enlarged. Movement of the ultrasound probe over this region frequently produces discomfort. Other tests that your doctor might obtain are a CAT scan or an MRI of this region. Just as with prostatitis, cultures of seminal vesicle secretions or semen are obtained and antibiotics are prescribed based upon any microorganisms that are identified.

Treatment for seminal vesiculitis is quite similar to treatment for prostatitis. Here's a list of some treatment approaches:

* **Conservative therapy**. Warm baths; pelvic floor relaxation techniques; muscle relaxants.

* **Antibiotic therapy**. Administered for long periods of time when infection has been identified.

* **Pain medications**. Ranging from nonsteroidal anti-inflammatory medications to narcotic therapy.

* **Injection of the seminal vesicles**. Injections into the seminal vesicles can be performed either with a TRUS guided needle or through a cystoscope. These injections can contain antibiotics or other agents that the clinician chooses, i.e., anesthetic agents. Experiences with this approach are anecdotal. No studies are available for review to determine the efficacy of this procedure.

* **Seminal vesiculectomy**. Several surgical approaches have been described to remove the seminal vesicles. This is really a last resort procedure used for patients with symptoms of infection and obvious abnormalities of the seminal vesicles that persist despite less aggressive therapy. When the seminal vesicles are removed, patients experience a "dry orgasm," i.e., little or no semen is seen. This obviously has an influence on fertility. Complications that can occur include injury to the nearby ureters or postoperative inability to attain an erection. As with injection therapy of the seminal vesicals, no literature exists documenting the benefits of this surgery in large numbers of patients. Those individuals most likely to improve from this surgery are those who have significant abnormalities of the seminal vesicals based upon MRI or CAT scan findings and documented infections in this area.

Prostate Cancer

Over the past ten to fifteen years prostate cancer has received an enormous amount of attention in medical and nonmedical circles. That's because this disease is now the most common cancer found in men. Thanks to increased awareness of the disease and active screening programs, prostate cancer is usually being diagnosed early on, and men are being cured.

But how does this relate to interstitial cystitis? Well, unfortunately, some men are not lucky enough to have their prostate cancer diagnosed early. When found in its later stages, prostate cancer can block the passage of urine. It can also extend into the bladder, causing the same type of irritative voiding symptoms seen with prostatic blockages and, yes, interstitial cystitis. Clinicians are advised to perform digital rectal examinations in all patients over forty years of age (and even younger if there's a family history of prostate cancer). Any area of hardness that's detected on the prostate examination could be related to a cancer and requires further evaluation.

Urologists usually recommend a blood test called PSA (Prostate Specific Antigen) on an annual basis in patients over the age of fifty (and younger if there's a family history of prostate cancer). The PSA test is often elevated in the presence of prostate cancer. The PSA test cannot "make" the diagnosis of prostate cancer because other problems such as prostatitis, prostate enlargement, and procedures such as cystoscopy also can cause PSA elevations. Some patients have no evidence of prostate cancer but have high PSA levels for unknown reasons. In any event, either an elevation of the PSA or an abnormality of the prostate found upon rectal exam warrants further evaluation.

Bladder Cancer

Bladder cancer is a disease more commonly seen in men than in women. In most instances, the first sign of bladder cancer is microscopic (the red blood cells can be seen only with a microscope) or visible blood in the urine. Pelvic pain associated with bladder cancer is unusual but, as with prostate cancer, it can be related to tumors that have deeply invaded the bladder wall or have extended to structures outside of the bladder.

Another form of bladder cancer known to cause irritative voiding symptoms or pain is called *carcinoma in situ* (CIS). Under the microscope, CIS appears as a tumor that has the tendency to spread rapidly; however, the tumor cells are only on the bladder's surface. Upon cystoscopy, this tumor appears as a red, velvety patch—pretty much identical in appearance to a Hunner's ulcer. That's why clinicians always will do a biopsy of the bladder surface when seeing unusual lesions like these.

The urine cytology test is a very useful noninvasive test for detecting bladder cancer. Cells lining the urinary tract normally shed into the urine, much like dandruff from the scalp. These cells are examined under a microscope specifically for any evidence of cancer. The sensitivity of urine cytology is highest for aggressive tumors (also called high-grade tumors) and CIS, tumor types commonly associated with irritative voiding symptoms.

Differences Between Men and Women in the Treatment of IC

Management strategies between male and female IC patients are generally the same; however, there can be subtle differences. Outlined below is a listing of some observations that we've made regarding these differences.

1. As was mentioned early in this chapter, men can have associated medical problems that result in symptoms similar to interstitial cystitis. Prostate problems, either prostatic enlargement or prostatitis, are by far the most common of these disorders. To achieve the best overall reduction in urinary symptoms, it's important to apply therapy to these problems along with IC therapy. For example, the male IC patient might have some improvement in symptoms on a course of Elmiron® and low-dose Elavil® but still have problems with a poor force of the urine stream. Further evaluation might reveal that the poor urine flow is due to a combination of prostatic enlargement and pelvic floor muscle spasm (a problem frequently associated with IC). In this case, additional therapy is warranted to deal with these other issues.

   One last point on the topic of a slow urine stream. If you have a poor urine flow, be very careful when taking over-the-counter cold remedies. Many of these medications work by "tightening up" blood vessels in the nose, thereby decreasing the amount of nasal stuffiness. Unfortunately, these medications also tighten up the muscles in the region of the bladder neck, resulting in a further restriction of the urine flow. Antihistamines also can cause difficulties with the passage of urine. Taking these types of medication has resulted in many a man making his way to the emergency room, unable to pass his urine. This is a condition called *acute urinary retention* and requires the passage of a urethral catheter to relieve the blockage. As you can well imagine, these men are not too comfortable in this situation. How do you know which over-the-counter medication might result in this problem? Look at the back of the medication box. The box for medications like these usually will recommend consulting your doctor if you are known to have prostate problems. Common ingredients of the medications that can lead to further urinary difficulties include: pseudoephedrine, phenylpropanolamine, phenylephrine, chlorpheniramine, diphenhydramine, and brompheramine. If your nose is really stuffy, it's probably safer to use a nasal spray—although even these medications can (rarely) cause problems if the medication is absorbed into the bloodstream. You should also be aware that some of the medications that we use in the management of interstitial cystitis can slow bladder function, leading to further problems (see chapter 5, Oral Medications).

2. When pelvic floor dysfunction occurs in the male IC patient, it often causes severe pain. In our experience, the pain is often worse than in female patients. Perhaps this is related to the larger and more bulky pelvic muscles often encountered in male patients. The symptoms that are usually the most disconcerting are those relating to pain that occurs during or shortly after orgasm. The pain can be so intense that many of these patients avoid sexual intercourse altogether. The location of the pain varies. Examples of typical complaints are as follows:

    *   Throbbing or burning pain at the tip of the penis. Touching the penis in this region rarely causes additional pain. That's because the pain doesn't actually originate there. The pain usually comes from deep in the pelvis, in the region of the prostate or pelvic floor muscles.

    *   Pain all along the shaft of the penis, also often described as throbbing or burning.

    *   Pain around the anus or perineum. This can be worsened even further by associated constipation.

    *   Aggressive care is needed in these instances. Forms of therapy that can be helpful include:

        *   Frequent warm baths. Sitz baths can also be helpful.

        *   Avoidance of constipation.

* Avoidance of sitting for long periods of time (longer than twenty minutes).

* Use of muscle relaxants.

* Use of nonsteroidal anti-inflammatory medications.

* Use of physical therapy.

* Use of biofeedback and electrical stimulation therapy of the pelvic floor.

* Use of alternative strategies (like acupuncture, meditation, yoga, etc.). Yoga seems to be particularly helpful to many patients.

Many of these techniques are described elsewhere in this text.

3. One final bit of strong advice. Don't jump to very invasive forms of care such as surgery first. Start with conservative strategies like those just described above. It's easy to stop taking a pill or to hold off on biofeedback treatments if you feel that they're not helpful or are worsening your symptoms. On the other hand, a surgical procedure is usually difficult if not impossible to undo. Over the past several years, we've seen several patients who have gone the surgical route and later regretted their decision. Whenever you are contemplating surgery, it's a very good idea to get a second opinion.

Chapter **8**

Surgery and the Interstitial Cystitis Patient

This chapter will focus on the many forms of surgical care available to the interstitial cystitis (IC) patient. The procedures that we'll discuss range from those performed in the office to the most aggressive forms of surgical therapy such as bladder removal (fortunately, a very rarely performed surgery for IC). In general, surgical procedures, particularly the more invasive ones, are used when simpler forms of care (such as dietary changes, oral or intravesical medications) fail.

Minimally Invasive Procedures

Minimally invasive procedures are frequently performed in the office setting with special surgical devices that do not require large incisions. There is less postoperative pain associated with these procedures than with open surgery and a faster recovery time.

Urethral Dilatation

Urethral dilation is a procedure usually performed in the office setting. Urethral dilations are sometimes used in the management of a condition called *urethral syndrome*. The procedure and its indications are discussed in detail in chapter 4, Medical Conditions Associated with Interstitial Cystitis.

Bladder Hydrodistention Under Anesthesia

Hydrodistention of the bladder is a common procedure performed to help establish a diagnosis of IC. It is discussed in chapter 1, Interstitial Cystitis 101: The Basics. One potential benefit of the procedure is that about 30-60 percent of patients will have some symptom improvement postoperatively. It seems that the patients who derive the most symptomatic benefit from bladder hydrodistention are those who have small bladders. If you undergo a hydrodistention, don't expect to feel better at first. In fact, most patients have a worsening of their IC symptoms for one to three weeks after the procedure. This is usually managed with pain medications and a urinary anesthetic. Recently, we have been instilling an "anesthetic cocktail" into the patients' bladders after hydrodistention (see chapter 6, Medications Introduced into the Bladder). They seem to wake up with less discomfort in the recovery room this way.

Complications of hydrodistention are rare but include the following:

* **Urinary infection**. This is an unusual problem since most doctors give patients an antibiotic at the time of the procedure. Even without an antibiotic, infection is unusual.

* **Bleeding**. Most patients will have some blood seen in their urine after the hydrodistention. Usually patients are told to drink lots of water and to avoid any strenuous activity for a few days. It's important to have been taken off blood thinner medications like aspirin or Coumadin® before the procedure (under the supervision of your medical doctor) because these agents increase the likelihood of postoperative bleeding problems. Despite excellent control of bleeding in the operating room, bleeding sometimes can recur, necessitating a return to the operating room.

* **Bladder rupture**. The bladder is exposed to a fairly high pressure of fluid during the hydrodistention process. The potential for the bladder to burst open is present, but fortunately this problem is very rare. That's because of the bladder's remarkable elasticity. Patients who have a decrease in

their bladder's elasticity—those patients with small, scarred bladders—are at a higher risk for this occurrence. Bladder rupture is also uncommon because the bladder is usually filled directly through the cystoscope. That means the bladder surface is being watched at all times during the filling process. At the first sign of any problem, the hydrodistention is terminated. Nevertheless, a sudden bladder rupture is possible. If a bladder rupture occurs, a catheter is usually left in the bladder for a few days. This allows time for healing and prevents urine from leaking outside the bladder. The doctor might want to perform an x-ray called a *cystogram* before removing the catheter. This test is performed to assure that no urine can leak out from the rupture area. Open surgical repair is almost never needed.

* **Urinary retention**. Some patients are unable to urinate after the procedure. This is almost always a short-lived problem but may necessitate having a catheter placed for a few days. The catheter is connected to a small bag that is attached to the leg (appropriately called a "leg bag"). The catheter is usually removed in the office setting. Urinary retention probably occurs because of a combination of factors such as postoperative spasm of the pelvic floor muscles and medications like narcotics, which are given for pain (narcotics decrease the bladder's ability to contract).

Certainly hydrodistention can be helpful to achieve symptom improvement for some patients, but its beneficial effects last on average only three months. We've noted that for those patients who feel better after hydrodistention, repeat procedures result in progressively less impressive symptom improvement. It's, therefore, probably best to use the procedure sparingly and in conjunction with other therapies.

Surgical Management of the Hunner's Ulcer

When interstitial cystitis was first described, the only patients who were diagnosed were those who had the "classical" form of the disease, those patients with small, shrunken bladders associated with Hunner's ulcers (regions of intense inflammation). Early reports suggested that surgical removal of these regions resulted in significant symptom improvement.

Resectoscopes

As surgical technology improved, resectoscopes (resect means to remove tissue) became available. These are specialized telescopes (similar to cystoscopes) that can be inserted into the bladder through the urethra; hence, no skin incisions are necessary. Resectoscopes have an attachment called a resecting loop that can "carve" away unwanted tissue. Removal of Hunner's ulcers using the resectoscope resulted in the same symptom improvement as the open surgical procedures.

Laser Therapy

Most recently, laser therapy has been directed at the Hunner's ulcer with similar success. The advantage of the laser is that tissue is burned away in a precise manner and creates only a small amount of residual scarring (as opposed to the significant scar tissue created by open surgery or resecting the entire region). Many types of lasers are available. The most common type used to treat Hunner's ulcers is the neodymium-YAG laser.

Laser therapy used to treat Hunner's ulcers is performed in the operating room under general or spinal anesthesia. The bladder is filled with irrigation fluid (usually sterile water) and the ulcers are inspected. As the laser energy is applied to the ulcers, they turn from a beefy red color to white. In the vast majority of patients, laser therapy of Hunner's ulcers achieves an excellent reduction in pain within twenty-four to forty-eight hours.

Our studies indicate an average decline in pain from 9.4 to 1.8 (on a 0–10 pain scale, 10 being the most severe pain), which was seen in the first twenty-four patients evaluated.

The biggest problem associated with the laser procedure is that the symptom relief doesn't usually last forever. Although we have patients who are symptom-free for well over three years, the majority of patients have symptom recurrence within six to nine months. When patients have recurrence of symptoms, repeat cystoscopy usually demonstrates new Hunner's ulcers, often in different regions than the previously treated ulcers. Re-treatment of these areas almost uniformly results in symptom improvement again—but who wants to go through another procedure every six to nine months? This is clearly a downside of the procedure. This relatively rapid reoccurrence of Hunner's ulcers was also seen in the original more invasive surgeries.

Our postoperative management after laser surgery has changed over the past few years. In the past, when patients went into remission after the procedure, they came off all or most of their other medications (like Elmiron®, Elavil®, and Atarax®). We now keep patients on these medications in the hope that continued use might delay ulcer recurrence. It should be kept in mind that no scientific study has been performed yet to substantiate this approach; however, these medications either protect the bladder surface or decrease inflammation and at least in theory they may help.

Complications of Laser Treatment

Laser treatment of the Hunner's ulcer usually proceeds uneventfully, but there is one major potential complication—i.e., bladder perforation. This means that a small hole can be made in the bladder during the procedure. The hole can be made even without the surgeon being aware of its existence. That's because the perforation starts off as a burn that goes all the way through the bladder wall.

Hunner's ulcers are usually found on the dome (the top) of the bladder. On the other side of that region of the bladder wall are the intestines. If a burn injury goes through the bladder wall, the intestines can be injured. They can leak their contents and peritonitis (infection of the abdominal lining) can take place. This problem doesn't occur right away. Patients who develop peritonitis in this setting may have worsening abdominal pain associated with fever for several days to weeks after the procedure. If this occurs, surgical exploration must be performed to identify the injury and to repair it. Fortunately, bladder perforations are rare.

Neurostimulation

In order to understand the technique of neurostimulation (also called neuromodulation), it's important to first understand a little about how the nervous system works, particularly the spine. Some of the functions that the spine performs include the following:

1. **Transmission of sensory information.** The spine has many very long nerves that transmit sensory information from the "peripheral" nerves (nerves from the skin, the bladder, and such) to the brain. Different types of sensations may travel through different areas within the spine.

2. **Coordinating motor function.** This means that the spine carries nerves that can cause a physical change in our bodies. An example of a physical change is the contraction of a muscle. A muscle contraction occurs by your brain sending signals directly down your spinal cord. These nerves then

communicate with other nerves (called motor neurons) that stimulate the desired muscle to contract.

Alternatively, the spine coordinates its sensory and motor functions through the brain. In this instance, your sensory nerves might tell you that a flower has a pleasant, fragrant smell. Your brain processes this information and your motor nerves then coordinate your movements closer to the flower for a deeper inhalation of its aroma.

In other instances, as with a spinal reflex, your brain isn't needed for a motor response. One example of this phenomenon is the "knee-jerk" reflex. In this situation, a region just below the knee is tapped. That tapping sensation is passed along nerves that go to the spinal cord. Those nerves then directly stimulate motor nerves within the spinal cord. The motor nerves then cause some of the leg muscles to contract causing the leg to jerk or twitch. Bladder function incorporates both reflex activity *and* input from the brain. As the bladder fills, nerves with special endings called stretch receptors send signals to the spinal cord. In the infant with a newly developing nervous system, a knee-jerk-like reflex occurs whereby the bladder contracts and the baby pees. As the nervous system develops, the brain begins to interact with this otherwise purely spinal process. The brain inhibits this reflex contraction on a moment-to-moment basis through nerves that run through the spinal cord.

Imagine this scene: You're at a movie theater. It's the climax of the movie, but that 32-ounce drink you purchased at the concession booth has started to affect your bladder. Your brain says that you need to hold off urinating just until this scene is over (this may elicit great pain for the IC patient). The brain sends stimulation down the spinal cord that inhibits the bladder contraction. The urge to urinate settles down somewhat. You can watch the movie for a few more minutes but the urge returns a few minutes later. This time, the urge may be greater, requiring an even higher degree of inhibition from the brain. Finally, you just have to run to the bathroom.

3. **The nerves within the spinal cord produce endorphins.** Endorphins are narcotics produced by the nervous system. They can result in pain relief and even a sense of euphoria.

The description above is a gross undersimplification of how the spinal cord works, but it will be useful to you in understanding the process of neurostimulation.

Neurostimulation, as its name implies, is a technique that stimulates the nervous system. The stimulation therapy is usually in the form of a low-voltage electrical current. The term neurostimulation is quite general, as it doesn't indicate exactly where the therapy is delivered. The nerve stimulation can occur at the level of the brain, the spinal cord, or even to the nerves of the structure to be treated (like the nerves that normally go to the bladder or are in the bladder itself).

Neurostimulation for the IC patient usually employs electrical energy that stimulates a *spinal nerve* (nerves that enter or exit the spinal cord). By doing so, all of the functions of the nerves described above can be altered. For example, neurostimulation might cause those nerves to secrete more endorphins, resulting in pain relief. They might also decrease their transmission of pain through the spine, or reduce the bladder's unwanted reflexive contractions.

Interstim® Therapy

Interstim therapy is a form of neurostimulation that was designed specifically to treat voiding problems. The Food and Drug Administration (FDA) originally approved the device for the treatment of urinary urge incontinence. Urgency incontinence is the unwanted leakage of urine due to uncontrolled bladder contractions. In 1999, Interstim therapy was further approved for the treatment of urinary retention (poor bladder emptying) and significant urinary urgency and frequency.

How the Interstim Works

The Interstim device employs a thin, floppy wire that is surgically placed beside nerves that participate in the functioning of the pelvic floor muscles. The specific area of wire placement is in the very lowest part of the back, called the *sacrum*. The nerve that is to be stimulated courses through one of several holes within the sacrum called the *sacral foramina*. The wire is placed beside the nerve at that point.

The wire is connected to a small pacemaker-like unit that provides a constant source of electrical stimulation. This unit looks just like a pacemaker for the heart, and just like a pacemaker, it runs on batteries that must be replaced every few years. The time between battery changes depends upon the energy level used for the particular patient.

Interstim therapy seems to work indirectly to improve bladder function. The nerves that control the function of the pelvic floor muscles are stimulated. Those are the muscles that must relax when you want to urinate. When you're not urinating, those muscles always have some resting tone (a moderate amount of muscle tension), just enough to avoid leakage. It's believed that stimulation of the pelvic floor muscles leads to a reflexive decrease in the bladder's ability to contract; hence it has the potential to stop those unwanted bladder contractions and associated incontinence.

Abnormal contractions of the pelvic floor muscles (pelvic floor dysfunction) occur in about 70 percent of IC patients (Moldwin and Mendelowitz 1993). Pelvic floor dysfunction can cause troubles with urinary frequency, urgency, pelvic pain, lower back pain, and constipation. The Interstim therapy unit seems to result in better pelvic floor muscle tone and a decrease in the symptoms often associated with pelvic floor dysfunction.

Pretesting with the Interstim

One very nice feature of Interstim therapy is the ability it provides to test the device out prior to a formal surgical implantation. After a local anesthetic is administered to the lower back, a floppy wire is placed next to the desired nerve through a special needle. The wire then exits the back and is carefully taped in place. It's then connected to a "neurostimulator unit" that is clipped to the belt of your pants.

The electrical stimulation is adjusted to a comfortable level for the patient and if all goes well, it achieves the desired symptomatic improvement. The stimulator unit is left in place for a few days. If symptom improvement occurs and continues, the patient is a candidate for a formal surgical implantation of the device. The testing phase is virtually without complications. The only problem that occasionally arises is some discomfort from the wire where it comes in contact with the skin. A skin infection can occur at the site where the wire exits the skin, but this is rare. The biggest problem with the testing phase is the potential for the wire to move out of position. Remember, there aren't any stitches to hold it in place—only tape. That means that the patient can do no significant bending of the back during the few days of testing.

In the event that the patient has a good response to the Interstim device, he or she becomes a candidate for surgical implantation in the operating room. In this case, an incision is made in the lower back. A very sophisticated wire that can deliver electrical stimulation at varying levels along its surface is sutured in place. Another small incision is made in the upper portion of the buttocks. The stimulator unit is then placed within the fat of that region and the wire is then connected to the unit.

Interstim Results

Results of Interstim therapy for urinary urgency-frequency after twelve months, reported by Medtronic (the company that designed the therapy), are as follows: Of thirty-three patients with implanted units, 33 percent had a reduction of voids by 50 percent or more. Thirty-one percent reduced their urinary frequency to the "normal" range (four to seven voids per day). Eighty-two percent became able to hold more urine in their bladders with each void.

Although the Interstim device can control the symptoms of urinary urgency and frequency for many patients, it doesn't seem to be as effective at pain management (although there are exceptions). Also about 20 percent of patients who have a "successful" testing phase have a suboptimal response when the device in finally implanted. Some complications of this surgical procedure include the following:

1. **Migration of the stimulator wire.** Even though the wire is sutured in place against the bone of the sacrum, in some instances the wire can move. (Movement of the wire by 1/16th of an inch, in some cases, can cause the system to become ineffective.) Reoperation may be needed in these instances.

2. **Wound infection.** This is a rare problem but when it does occur, it necessitates removal of the device. Infection of the bone (osteomyelitis) is even less common. When it occurs, long courses of antibiotic therapy usually are needed.

3. **The development of new pain.** This might require altering the settings of the neurostimulator unit. Changing the setting can be done by using a specially designed magnet.

4. **Pain at the site where the neurostimulator is placed.** This is a fairly common problem associated with Interstim therapy, occurring in about 15 percent of patients.

In general, most difficulties associated with Interstim therapy can be resolved with medications or reprogramming (using the reprogramming magnet). Sometimes, these issues simply resolve by themselves without any specific medical intervention. Nevertheless, about 33 percent of patients will need additional surgery to correct some problem associated with this system. Those problems usually relate to pain associated with the unit or misplacement of the neurostimulator wire.

In summary, neurostimulation using the Interstim system can be potentially helpful at alleviating symptoms of urinary urgency and frequency, but it has not been found to be as useful in the management of pain. It should be considered for therapy only when other less aggressive therapies have failed. If you or your physician is interested in this form of therapy, Medtronic recently has produced some very informative pamphlets about the Interstim system for patients. The pamphlets are quite detailed and very candid about the indications and possible complications associated with this new technology. Medtronic's phone number is (800) 328-0810; their web site is www.medtronic.com.

Other Neurostimulation Units

Another neurostimulation device produced by Advanced Neuromodulation Systems (ANS) has been useful in the treatment of chronic pain. This is a more complex device than the Interstim Unit and needs to be placed by a neurosurgeon.

The Per Q SANS (Stoller Afferent Nerve Stimulator) unit (UroSurge, Coralville, IA) is a newly FDA-approved device for the treatment of urinary urgency and frequency (as well as for urinary urgency incontinence). The device works by stimulating a nerve just above the ankle with a special needle. The needle is connected to an electrical stimulator unit. Therapy is applied once a week for twelve weeks. FDA trials have demonstrated a 71 percent success rate, success being defined as at least a 25 percent reduction in daytime or nighttime urinary frequency.

Other Neurological Procedures

Nerves have been surgically cut or destroyed at multiple levels in the nervous system with the hope that the symptoms of IC would abate. In many instances, immediate symptom improvement was attained. Unfortunately, long-term follow-up has shown a high rate of symptom recurrence. This issue plus a high rate of surgical complications has led most clinicians to abandon these procedures.

Urinary Diversion

It seems as if the urine itself may be the cause of many symptoms for the IC patient. Certain chemicals in the urine appear to irritate the bladder surface thereby stimulating the desire to urinate and causing pain. The bladder stretching while it fills with urine can also result in these symptoms. These facts have led us to ask these questions: What would happen if urine could exit the bladder as soon as it entered or, even better, what would happen if we could get the urine out of the body without it having to pass through the bladder (urinary diversion)? Could there be a decrease in symptoms? Just as important, how would we do it? Here are some procedures that have been developed to deal with these issues.

The Urethral Catheter

The urethral catheter was discussed in chapter 6, Medications Introduced into the Bladder, and is included in this chapter as a procedure that can be used to divert the flow of urine. Placement of the catheter is not a surgical procedure. The specific type of catheter that is used in this instance is called the Foley catheter. This catheter has a balloon at its tip (filled with water) that prevents it from slipping out of the bladder. Any urine that enters the bladder from the kidneys will pass through the catheter and outside the body. Therefore, the bladder never fills up.

The catheter is usually attached to a "leg bag" during the daytime. This is a small bag that straps onto the leg and collects urine. During sleeping hours, the catheter is attached to a large bag that hangs from the side of the bed. The large bag is used at night so that the patient doesn't need to keep emptying the bag at night. Additionally, having the bag at the side of the bed allows urine to flow with gravity away from the bladder. If a leg bag were to be used at night, the bladder and the bag would both be at the same level and the force of gravity would not be called into play. Thus urine could easily back up from the bag into the bladder. It's important to have a "one-way" flow of urine to the collection bag in order to prevent any bacteria that might be growing in the bag from gaining entrance into the bladder.

The Foley catheter can be helpful for the patient who is having significant flare in symptoms and is going to the bathroom continually. It allows the bladder a little time to "rest." On the other hand, the catheter can irritate the bladder and cause more symptoms for the IC patient. It's hard to know what will happen until the catheter is put into place. In our experience, the Foley catheter can be helpful for the first few days, sometimes even a week or two. After that, it begins to irritate the bladder and patients almost always want it out.

A urinary tract infection is another problem that can occur while the catheter is in place. The longer the catheter is in the bladder, the higher the chance of developing an infection.

Many IC patients have urethral pain. This can makes Foley catheter placement difficult from the start. That leads us to the suprapubic tube (also called the suprapubic catheter).

The Suprapubic Catheter

The suprapubic catheter, as its name implies, is a tube that drains the bladder directly through the lower abdomen just above (*supra* means "above") the pubic bone. The patient does not need to be hospitalized because the suprapubic tube can be placed in the doctor's office under local anesthesia. A small incision (about ¼ inch) is created in the skin. Then, a special needle, usually accompanied by the catheter, is advanced directly into the bladder. The correct position is verified when urine is returned through the tube. The needle is removed and the catheter is left in place.

After about three to four weeks, the tube can be changed, again in the doctor's office. Tube changes are not performed prior to that time because the tract would immediately close down, preventing the new catheter from being placed. The biggest problem for the IC patient with regard to suprapubic tube placement is the need for a full bladder during the procedure.

The empty bladder normally sits low in the pelvis, behind the pubic bone. (Clinicians can tell your bladder is empty when they push on the lower abdomen and can easily feel the top of your pubic bone.) If the bladder is not full when the needle comes through, other organs such as the intestines may be punctured, leading to serious complications.

Another reason that the bladder needs to be full is that the special needle has an easy job puncturing a tense bladder. The needle has a much more difficult time puncturing a floppy bladder. What does this all mean for the IC patient? It means that if you're planning on follow through with such a procedure, your doctor might want to place the tube under anesthesia in the operating room. That way the bladder can be filled to its capacity without any discomfort to you.

The suprapubic tube is usually placed in the patient who needs to have urinary diversion on a chronic basis or who has severe urethral pain when a urethral catheter is placed. It's usually easier to care for than a urethral catheter and has fewer associated long-term complications. However, as with a urethral catheter, the suprapubic tube can be associated with urinary tract infections.

One common problem is the leakage of some urine around the tube. The suprapubic tube can irritate the bladder in the same way a urethral catheter can. If it causes more pain, it can be easily removed in the office. The passage from the bladder to the skin usually closes off within a day or two.

Invasive Surgical Procedures (Open Surgery)

As the name implies, these procedures are more invasive and are almost always performed as a last resort. They are performed in the operating room with a hospital stay of approximately five to ten days, and a convalescence of about six weeks.

Procedures to Remove Almost All of the Bladder

Many an IC patient has said, "I just wish that I could have a new bladder." Well, a surgical procedure was developed that did just about that. The procedure was called the "supratrigonal cystectomy and cystoplasty." In English, this means that almost the entire bladder is removed, leaving only the base (called the trigone) and the urethra. A segment of intestine is then reshaped and attached to the remaining base to create a new larger bladder. (See figure 11.)

This might sound like a great idea but, unfortunately, many patients experienced no relief of pain after the procedure. That's probably because much of the IC patient's pain is derived from the bladder base. Additionally, the newly created bowel-bladder did not function exactly like a normal bladder. About 30 percent of patients had new bladders that didn't empty effectively. Those patients had to then begin a course of intermittent catheterization, a procedure where the patient catheterizes him or herself four to six times a day to remove the urine.

Of course, lots of patients with IC have very sensitive urethras, which made catheterization a very painful process. The important message to take away here is that the supratrigonal cystectomy is a surgical procedure rarely indicated for the patient with interstitial cystitis. It is contemplated only for the patient who has demonstrated the following:

1. Has had a poor response to all other therapies.

2. Has a bladder that has shrunken with scar tissue to walnut size.

3. Does not have pelvic pain as a major problem.

4. Can perform intermittent self-catheterization, if needed.

Only a small number of IC patients are candidates for this surgery. Of those patients, an extremely small number meet the criteria that are described here.

Diverting the Flow of Urine Above the Bladder (Supravesical Diversion)

Catheters designed to remove urine rapidly from the bladder can sometimes relieve bladder pain (see "Minimally Invasive Procedures" above), but they are far from perfect. They can cause a lot of irritation all by themselves. Additionally, although they can prevent

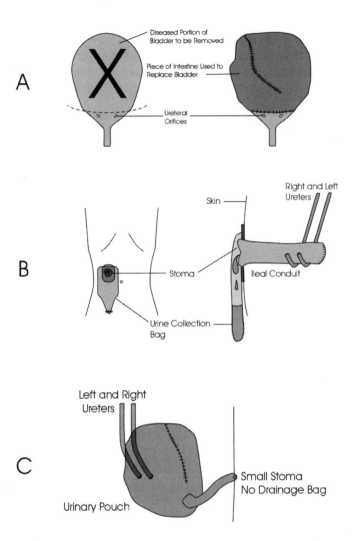

Figure 11. Various Types of Urinary Diversion. (A) Supratrigonal cystectomy and cystoplasty. (B) Ileal conduit. (C) Urinary "pounc."

urine from building up in the bladder, the bladder surface is still exposed to urine prior to the urine exiting via the tube. Some clinicians believe that complete diversion of urine from the bladder is needed to attain the best reduction in symptoms. This comes at a big cost—major surgery.

Today, most surgeons agree that if such surgery is contemplated, it should be combined with cystectomy (complete removal of the bladder) to achieve the best results. Let's go over some of these procedures with their associated complications.

The Ileal Conduit

The ileal conduit (see figure 11B) is considered by most urologists to be the "gold standard" procedure used to divert urine. The procedure uses a short segment of the small intestine, called the ileum. The tubes that normally carry urine from the kidneys to the bladder (the ureters) are separated from the bladder (the bladder is usually removed) and connected to this small piece of intestine. One of the ends of the intestine is sutured closed. The other end exits the skin as a "stoma" (an artificially created small opening).

The urine drains through the stoma into a collection bag. As the bag fills, the urine is drained from the bag into the toilet several times per day. With the ileal conduit there is no restriction on physical activities. Younger patients and some older patients frequently have concerns about their self-image with this form of therapy. Psychological counseling and counseling with an enterostomal therapist must be considered *before* this surgery is performed. Overall, once patients are relieved of their symptoms, they rapidly accommodate to the stoma.

Of all the forms of urinary diversion, the ileal conduit is associated with the fewest complications. These can be broken down to early (during surgery and up to three months after surgery) and late complications (occurring later than three months after surgery). Some of these complications are discussed below:

Early Complications

1. Problems associated with anesthesia.

2. Hemorrhage.

3. Poor survival of the piece of ileum. The blood supply of the short piece of intestine can decrease in the postoperative period, sometimes to the point where the tissue can't survive. In these instances, a new conduit must be created.

4. Infection.

5. The development of scar tissue (stricture) at the point where the urine enters the ileal conduit. This can cause a blockage of urine and usually requires some form of surgical repair.

6. Leakage of urine outside the conduit and into the abdominal cavity. This is another problem that often requires surgical repair.

Late Complications

1. Scarring of the conduit to the point where the urine has a hard time getting into the bag. This usually occurs at the skin level and is called stomal stenosis.

2. Blockage of urine where it enters the conduit (see number five in "Early Complications" above).

3. Kidney infections associated with a decline in kidney function.

As you can see, there are complications that can occur with these types of procedures, many requiring another operation. In these procedures, along with the urinary diversion, the bladder is usually removed for the following two reasons:

1. Left in place, the bladder is an empty sac with no fluid running through it. It is, therefore, a set-up for the development of infection.

2. One cannot state with any degree of certainty that the bladder pain is caused only by urine running over its surface. It is just as likely that the pain derived from the bladder is completely independent of urine flow. Therefore, most surgeons will perform cystectomy (bladder removal) along with the urinary diversion.

The Catheterizable Bowel Pouch

Many patients do not like the idea of wearing an external bag to collect their urine. In response to this issue, new surgical procedures have been developed to create an "internal bag," made of intestine, that can be emptied several times a day. (See figure 11C.) When performing this type of surgery, a much larger piece of intestine is employed than that used for the ileal conduit.

Many types of procedures have been described, all using different portions of the bowel. Essentially, the segment of intestine is opened, then reshaped to create a large pouch. Like the ileal conduit, the ureters are connected to the pouch. Finally, another narrow segment of intestine is used to connect the pouch to the skin. Often the opening where the urine comes out is created right in the belly button. The skin opening is very small when compared to the stoma (opening) that is created for the ileal conduit. A urethral catheter is advanced into this small skin opening four to six times or more each day in order to remove urine from the pouch.

Overall, this sounds a lot easier to live with than the ileal conduit, but there are some down sides, as described below:

1. The creation of a urinary pouch takes longer to perform in the operating room. The cystectomy and creation of the pouch can take five to eight hours or more.

2. The hospital stay is often longer and the patient leaves the hospital with a large tube that drains the pouch. When patients go home, they need to instill fluid through this tube several times a day. This procedure clears out mucus that is produced by the pouch. Eventually, the pouch slows down its production of mucus and the tube is then removed in the doctor's office.

3. There's a lot more stitching that must be done to create a pouch as opposed to the ileal conduit. This means that there's a higher chance for urine to leak out of the pouch and cause problems.

4. A urinary pouch shouldn't be performed in patients who have poor kidney function because the kidney function could worsen after the pouch is created.

5. The narrow piece of intestine that comes out onto the skin should not leak urine. In some cases, leakage does occur. This may require surgical revision.

6. In rare instances, it becomes difficult to empty the pouch because the small stoma becomes difficult to catheterize. This also might require surgical revision.

7. Some IC patients who have undergone this procedure have developed "pouch pain." Some people have termed this "pouchitis." Biopsies of the pouch in some patients have demonstrated inflammation of the pouch wall but other investigations have shown that inflammation is a normal response of the bowel when exposed to urine (MacDermott, Charpied, Tesluk, and Stone 1990).

Recommendations Regarding Bladder Removal

Removal of the bladder is considered only when all other conservative forms of therapy have failed. Keep in mind that there are many reasons, apart from IC, for an individual to experience pelvic pain. It is therefore extremely important for the clinician to identify as best as possible that the pelvic pain does indeed originate from the bladder—before proceeding with bladder removal.

Although it is possible to simply divert the urine (using a pouch or ileal conduit) and leave the bladder in place, most clinicians tend to stay away from this approach because of the high likelihood of continued bladder pain and the possibility of infections occurring in the remaining unused bladder.

Likewise, most IC specialists are shying away from the supratrigonal cystectomy (removal of almost all of the bladder, leaving the bladder base behind; then replacing the portion of bladder removed with a piece of intestine) because of the high rate of persistent symptoms. The only type of patient who is usually considered for this surgery has little associated pain and a small contracted bladder (a very rare IC patient).

When it comes down to the decision between an ileal conduit or an internal pouch, we usually recommend an ileal conduit unless the patient has an aversion to using an external urine collection bag. The reason for this recommendation is the possibility of developing pain within the pouch. This appears to be a relatively rare event, but when it does occur, it can be quite disconcerting for the patient. This is not to say that the creation of a pouch is a bad decision. It just means that an ileal conduit is associated with fewer problems.

Chapter 9

Sex and Interstitial Cystitis

Making love is a normal part of human experience. Unfortunately, it's a part that is often denied to the interstitial (IC) patient due to associated pain. This can take a terrible psychological toll on relationships where the loss of sexual activity extends to the loss of any type of physical interaction—this often starts a downhill progression that ends in couples breaking up or just drifting apart. This is a problem that must be addressed early on in the management of IC, and is more commonly seen in the female patient. In this short chapter, some of the causes of pain and management strategies for dealing with it are discussed.

Pain Associated with Sexual Intercourse

There are many reasons that you can develop *dyspareunia* (pain with sexual intercourse). Many of the causes are treated differently, so let's break them down into two basic groups:

1. **Entry Dyspareunia.** This means that the pain occurs at the opening of the vagina. Some problems that can cause this type of pain include the following:

   * **Atrophic vaginitis.** This is caused by estrogen loss and is therefore most commonly seen in postmenopausal women.

Estrogen replacement therapy might be recommended. Either oral replacements or local creams can be used.

* **Vaginitis**. This is an inflammation of the vagina, usually due to a fungal infection. It can cause severe irritation during sexual intercourse. These infections usually can be treated with either antifungal oral medications or creams.

* **Herpes or other lesions of the vulva**. Therapy is dependent on what type of lesion is detected.

* **Vulvodynia**. This problem is discussed in some detail in chapter 4, Medical Conditions Associated with Interstitial Cystitis. Briefly, vulvodynia means vulvar pain of unknown cause. Patients often describe penile entry feeling like dragging sandpaper across an open wound (with a little salt added in for good measure). Given this type of sensation, one can easily understand why sex would be out of the question.

* **Infection within the glands of the vulva**. Several glands found in this region can become infected. Sometimes the infection can be treated with antibiotics; in some cases, though, the infection must be treated surgically.

2. **Deep Dyspareunia**. This is the most common type of dyspareunia in the IC patient. The pain can come from several of the following sources:

* **Vaginal infections or lesions**.

* **Severe dryness of the vaginal lining**. This problem can be caused by estrogen loss. Psychological distress also can decrease the normally produced lubrication of this region.

* **Bladder pain**. The bladder is situated against the front portion of the vagina. Pressure from the penis in this region can cause pain, particularly when much of the pelvic pain originates in the bladder.

* **Pain from other pelvic abnormalities**. Examples of other diseases that can cause pelvic pain include endometriosis, ovarian diseases, pelvic infections, and diverticulitis of the colon. A careful medical evaluation is needed to exclude these possibilities.

* **Pain from the pelvic floor muscles**. This is one of the most common causes of pain associated with sexual

intercourse in the IC patient. Pelvic floor spasm occurs in approximately 70 percent of IC patients (see chapter 4). In some instances, the muscles of the pelvis can be so tight as to prevent the insertion of the penis. Then, a vicious cycle of muscle spasm is established as outlined below.

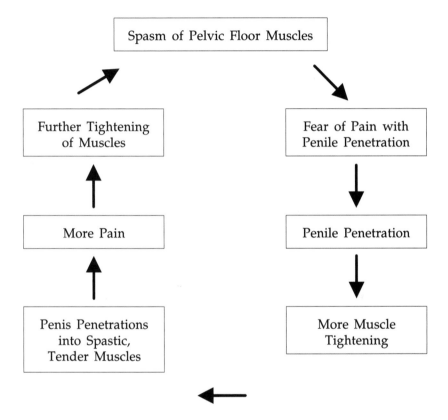

As you can see, the anticipation of pain causes more muscle spasm that often leads to even more pain. To make matters worse, the pain is intensified when the penis pushes into these hard, tender muscles.

It's important to remember that one or all of the above noted problems can be the cause of painful sexual intercourse. For example, the dyspareunia might vanish when receiving therapy for IC. If the urinary urgency, frequency, and pelvic pain subside, but the pain with intercourse persists, other issues such as vulvodynia or pelvic floor dysfunction might need to be addressed. Many of these problems have been discussed in other parts of this book. Please refer to the Index for more detailed information

General Management Principles

1. **Talk to your partner.** Difficulties with sexual relationships usually create frustration. The biggest mistake that you can make right from the beginning is to pretend that the problem doesn't exist. A "game plan" needs to be created that will deal with your needs as well as your partner's. If you need help discussing these issues, make sure that you speak to your medical caregiver about them. Other resources include psychologists and social workers who specialize in sexual dysfunction.

2. **Don't focus predominantly on vaginal penetration.** This may sound like a bit of a cop out, but it's stated for one simple reason. Making love goes far beyond the final act of penis going into vagina. It's a good idea to place a major focus upon foreplay including mutual full body massage with oils (often great for the fibromyalgia patient), deep kissing, fondling, oral-genital contact, etc. It's important to be creative keeping principle Number One in mind; that is, *talk to your partner.*

3. **Watch out for the effects of medication on orgasm.** Many medications used to treat IC can cause fatigue and/or a loss in sexual desire. Furthermore, some medications, most notably the antidepressants, can impair the ability to achieve orgasm. If you believe that this might be occurring, speak to your medical caregiver about it. Medications and/or their doses sometimes can be changed to deal with this problem.

4. **Go slow.** Many IC patients have terrible memories of painful sexual intercourse. Those memories are carried along each time they attempt to have sexual relations. As soon as the penis approaches the vagina, the pelvic floor muscles reflexively tighten as noted in the diagram above. The penis "hits" these areas and *Yikes! Severe Pain!* A substantial portion of the pain occurs because the penis is coming into contact with muscles that are in spasm. It is therefore very important to try as much as is possible to relax these muscles prior to and during penetration. That's easy to say but not always that easy to do. The best way to begin is to go slowly with both initial insertion of the penis and with thrusting. Reread the discussion of pelvic floor dysfunction in chapter 4. It reviews strategies to deal with this problem.

5. **Use lots of lubrication.** A lack of vaginal lubrication, no matter what the cause, will cause problems with achieving

penetration. It often also results in the inability to orgasm and causes further pain. There is absolutely no reason for this to be a problem. Multiple vaginal lubricants are available over-the-counter. There are even prescription lubricants available that have been combined with an anesthetic. These formulations can be especially helpful to the vulvodynia patient.

6. **Be in control.** This principle goes along with going slow. You need to know what to expect and the only way to accomplish this task is to call the shots. If you feel that thrusting can go deeper or faster, say so. If you're becoming irritated in the vulvar region, communicate this to your partner. You should also be in charge of choosing the most suitable sexual position.

7. **Find the right position for yourself.** There is no one sexual position that is correct for every couple. That's because there are multiple anatomical variations that factor into this equation. Some of these factors include the site of vulvar or vaginal tenderness; the angle of the vaginal vault; the size and curvature of the penis; and the weight of each partner. In general, the missionary position (man facing woman, man on top) causes discomfort for many female IC patients. That's probably because the penis is often deflected toward the bladder. Placing the woman on top usually affords better control. Other positions that seem to work better are vaginal penetration from the side or from behind. Again, it's important to experiment.

8. **Go one step at a time.** Don't make it a goal for either partner to orgasm while the penis is in the vagina (at least, not at first). To do so is often a set-up for disappointment. Rather, a step-wise approach to vaginal penetration is needed. For example, after foreplay, the penis can be slowly rubbed between the thighs near the vagina or against the clitoris/vaginal opening (add lots of lubrication). If this doesn't cause much discomfort, begin very superficial penetration (½-inch to 1-inch deep). This can be followed by deeper penetration depending upon symptoms. If some pain occurs, go back to more superficial contact or other forms of sexual stimulation. Don't stay focused upon vaginal entry! Going slowly in this manner also gives a better sense of control and hopefully helps to keep the pelvic muscles relaxed. Successful vaginal penetration is often a slow process for the IC patient. Don't assume that you'll be able to have deep

penetration, even if you go "step by step," in one sexual encounter. It may take five to ten or more efforts before anything close to satisfactory penetration occurs. In the meantime, as has been said before, don't focus only upon vaginal penetration. The other facets of the sexual encounter can be just as (or more) enjoyable.

9. **Avoid intercourse during flares.** There are times, often related to the menstrual cycle, that you can pretty much predict that sex is going to be a problem. The overall symptoms of IC begin to flare as manifested by an increase in urinary frequency and pelvic pain. These times often occur about one to two weeks before the menstrual flow. It is probably best to avoid sexual activity during these intervals since sexual intercourse can lead to a more intense flare in symptoms. It's important to note that other forms of sexual stimulation at these times usually *don't* cause a symptom flare.

10. **Take advantage of remissions.** We find that many patients who are feeling relatively well avoid sexual relations because they're afraid of starting up the symptoms again. This is certainly a possibility, but we still encourage a trial in most patients. As long as they don't "go for the gold" on their first encounter and take things slow (as outlined here), most patients do pretty well. When and if symptoms worsen after a sexual encounter, they usually settle down quickly.

11. **Take a warm bath after sex.** This can help relax the pelvic floor muscles after intercourse. It's also not a bad idea to take a bath *before* sexual activity. It's therapeutic for many patients and can be worked into sexual relations. Although the warmth soothes most patients, it may irritate others. If you have more discomfort from heat, applying a cold pack to the vulvar region will often make you more comfortable.

12. **Avoid urinary tract infections.** See chapter 4, Medical Conditions Associated with Interstitial Cystitis.

13. **Avoid using the diaphragm for contraception.** The diaphragm is associated with an increased risk of urinary tract infection. Additionally, many patients find that the device increases vaginal discomfort. The spermacide used with the diaphragm causes vaginal pain in some patients.

14. **Use vaginal dilators/biofeedback.** It sometimes helps to practice relaxing the vaginal vault. This can be accomplished

with the aid of an artificial penis (commonly called a "dildo"). Some of these items are sold with vibrator attachments. The vibrator units can be used for sexual stimulation but some patients complain that they actually worsen symptoms. Alternatively, medically prescribed silicon "vaginal dilators" can be used. The idea here is that a patient can slowly insert the dilator or artificial penis into the vagina (with lots of lubrication) and learn to relax her pelvic floor muscles around it. The nice aspect of this approach is that the patient is in total control of insertion. Insertion of the dilator, like penile penetration, is performed in a step-wise fashion. Biofeedback is another method of gaining control of the muscles of the pelvic floor. A "probe" is placed into the vagina and muscle tightness is seen on a computer screen. Using this information, patients can slowly learn to decrease muscle tension in this area.

15. **A note about the male IC patient.** Pelvic floor dysfunction is one of the most common causes of pain with sexual intercourse. It is often manifested by pain at the time of orgasm/ejaculation. The muscles responsible for the ejaculation of the semen need to contract vigorously to propel the semen forward. When the muscles are tender from the start, muscle contraction often results in more discomfort. In our experience, intensive therapy for pelvic floor dysfunction is often helpful.

16. **Read more about the subject.** *A Woman's Guide to Overcoming Sexual Fear and Pain* (Goodwin and Agronin 1997) is an excellent reference and guide on this topic.

Final Comments

There are a great number of patients who persist with dyspareunia despite extraordinary efforts to deal with this problem. If you're one of these patients and are reading this chapter, you probably still have a desire for intimacy with your partner—*so don't just drop it!* Go back to principles Numbers One and Two (talk to your partner and don't focus predominantly on vaginal penetration); work out methods of sexual satisfaction that don't concentrate on vaginal penetration). Similarly, intimacy goes far beyond the bedroom. Simple physical contacts like holding hands while walking, stroking your partner's arm while watching television, or a periodic kiss on the back of the neck are great ways to keep your relationship tuned up and running smoothly.

Chapter 10

Conservative Therapies for Interstitial Cystitis

This chapter reviews forms of treatment that have nothing to do with traditional medications or surgical procedures. Patients can administer some of these therapies themselves. Other forms of care involve practitioners other than doctors or nursing specialists. Unfortunately, some of the topics discussed in this chapter have no clinical research to substantiate their efficacy; however, their continued use by interstitial cystitis (IC) patients and anecdotal good responses merits mention here.

Dietary Changes

Diet has an influence on the symptoms of IC in over 50 percent of patients. This being the case, dietary modification has become one of the first and surprisingly effective forms of therapy for many sufferers. There are numerous "IC diets" that you can find on the Internet or in other published literature—but the essential fact is that *not every IC patient responds to the same diet.*

We've seen many an IC patient try to eliminate every food that "might" worsen their symptoms. Often the end result is continued symptoms and some serious malnutrition. The key to establishing an "eat this food and I'll pay the price later" list is to experiment. Once you've established that a particular food causes symptoms, then it would probably be a good idea to eliminate it entirely from your diet.

Let's start out with the foods and beverages that seem to most frequently cause symptom flares.

Foods That May Cause a Worsening of IC Symptoms

* Citrus fruits (oranges, grapefruits, lemons) apples, apricots, avocados, bananas, cantaloupes (you may be able to eat other melons), cranberries, grapes, nectarines, peaches, plums, rhubarb, strawberries

* Caffeinated beverages (Watch out. Many decaffeinated brands still have plenty of caffeine.)

* Chocolate

* Alcoholic beverages (particularly red wine)

* Tomatoes and tomato sauces

* Spicy foods

* Carbonated beverages

Other foods, food additives, or beverages that might worsen symptoms include the following:

* Aspartame (Nutrasweet), saccharine, foods with artificial colors, monosodium glutamate (MSG), citric acid

* Cheeses (except American, cottage, cream, ricotta)

* Sour cream

* Yogurt

* Chicken livers

* Corned beef and other smoked meats

* Pickled herring

* Vinegar

* Salad dressing

* Mayonnaise

* Lentils, lima beans, fava beans, soy beans

* Nuts (almonds, pine nuts, and peanuts are okay)

* Onions

* Raisins, cranberries, prunes

* Rye and sourdough bread

* Soy sauce

* Tea (Some herbal teas are okay; others can be a problem; it's hard to tell which will have a negative effect.)

Adapted with permission from Gillespie, *You Don't Have to Live with Cystitis!* (1986) and ICA Internet site—www.ichelp.org.

The question for you now is this: "How do I *experiment* with my diet to suit my needs?"

The simplest approach is to eliminate all of the possible offenders noted above for a week or two; then introduce them back into your diet, one by one. It's very helpful to keep a log of the foods that you reintroduce and to record the time when you reintroduce them. If a particular food or beverage is going to cause difficulties, it will likely be evident within six to twelve hours (you'll have a worsening of symptoms). The tricky part here is what to do when you're not certain that a food caused a problem for you. In these situations, just take it out of your diet for a few days and then reintroduce it again. Keep on repeating this process until you're reasonably sure that a particular item is a problem or not.

In many instances, the effect of food on symptoms also depends on how much you ingest. Sometimes it's possible to "get away" with taking a very small portion of a food that would otherwise cause a symptom flare. Figuring out how much you can eat without paying the price also takes some experimentation.

Food Acidity and the Symptoms of IC

Many IC patients report that acidic foods worsen their symptoms. (Why this occurs is unclear because many acidic foods don't result in a significant change in the acidity of the urine.) Apart from simply avoiding these foods and beverages altogether, strategies that seem to help patients deal with this problem include the following:

* Try Prelief, a "deacidifier." This tasteless additive is sprinkled on food. Using this agent, some patients report that they can eat foods that would otherwise cause a flare in their symptoms. Prelief is sold as an over-the-counter food additive. You can find more information through the web site www.prelief.com or by calling 800-994-4711.

* Try baking soda. Baking soda can neutralize acids. Drinking a glass of water with the addition of ½ teaspoon of baking soda three times per day may improve symptoms of urgency and frequency. Patients with high blood pressure should be careful to avoid using too much baking soda because of the high sodium content (high sodium can cause fluid retention and worsening of high blood pressure).

* Try potassium citrate. This is a standard form of medical therapy to decrease the acidity of the urine. Potassium citrate sometimes can cause stomach upset. Special preparations like Urocit-K® (a prescription drug) are often better tolerated.

* An excellent cookbook specifically produced for the IC patient is called *A Taste of the Good Life: A Cookbook for the Interstitial Cystitis Diet*, by Beverly Laumann.

Special Food Sensitivities

Allergies to certain foods may provoke a flare of IC or cause other bodily complaints, from migraine headaches to hives to abdominal cramping. The presence of yeast sensitivity also has been discussed as a possible cause of IC symptoms with anecdotal reports of symptom improvement on yeast-free diets (check this out at the ICA web site, www.ichelp.org). If you suspect that you have a food allergy, it might be helpful to speak with an allergist or nutritionist.

Fluid Intake

Many IC patients cut down on their fluid intake in the hope that their urinary frequency will settle down. Yes, it's true that *less in* will mean *less out*, but to rely on chronic dehydration is an unhealthy practice. Dehydration concentrates all of the noxious agents in the urine, agents that may worsen the symptoms of interstitial cystitis (particularly the pain component).

The recommendation for most IC patients is to increase their fluid intake—the best fluid to use is water. The most common question asked about fluid intake is, how much water should I drink? The answer will vary from person to person and depends upon the person's size, age, kidney function (which is usually perfectly normal), and level of physical activity. Finding the right amount of fluid to drink is definitely a balancing act. Taking too little can worsen symptoms; taking too much will have you peeing too much.

Don't Forget the Bowels!

A high percentage of IC patients have either irritable bowel syndrome (characterized by abnormal spasms of the small and/or large intestine giving rise to abdominal pain and alternating diarrhea and constipation) or chronic constipation. These problems frequently worsen the symptoms of IC. They absolutely must be evaluated and treated in order to see the best improvement in your symptoms. A high fiber diet as well as the use of psyllium (Metamucil®, Fibercon®) can be helpful. Mild laxatives and enemas may be needed at times as directed by your medical caregiver.

Biofeedback and Electrical Stimulation (E-stim) Therapy

Biofeedback is a learning technique the goal of which is to obtain better control over a bodily function. To accomplish this, the individual receives immediate information regarding the function by some form of medical technology. A good example of how biofeedback works is seen in the treatment of tension headache.

Tension headaches are caused by the spasm of muscles located on the front and side of the head and jaw. Electrodes (similar to those used for EKGs) are placed on the skin overlaying these muscles. Muscle contraction creates electrical activity that is picked up by the electrodes just as an EKG picks up the heartbeat. The more intense the muscle contraction, the more electrical energy is created. Then, information regarding the intensity of muscle contraction is "fed back" to the patient.

The feedback information is usually displayed graphically on a computer screen but it could just as easily be converted to another form, like sound. By receiving this information, the individual can learn to relax her or his muscles more effectively and, hopefully, achieve better control over their headaches.

Biofeedback and the Urinary Tract

As far as the urinary tract is concerned, biofeedback has been used for several years in the management of urinary incontinence (see the section on pelvic floor dysfunction in chapter 4). A probe (with electrodes on its surface) is placed in the vagina (or the rectum in the male). Pelvic floor muscle activity is displayed graphically on a monitor that the patient views. Electrodes are also placed over the abdominal muscles to detect their activity. Patients are then asked to tighten the muscles of the pelvic floor. Initially, many patients incorrectly contract their abdominal muscles rather than their pelvic muscles; but with the help of the feedback information they learn to contract and relax the muscles of the pelvic floor exclusively. The electrode doesn't only detect that the muscles are contracting. It also displays the force of the contraction as represented by the muscles' electrical activity. As patients continue the process, they gain muscle strength and tone in that region. Patients practice contracting their pelvic muscles on a daily basis at home. These exercises are often called "Kegels," named after the gynecologist who originally described them, Dr. A. H. Kegel.

Many probes used for biofeedback also can deliver electrical energy to the muscles and nerves of the pelvic floor, a process called *electrical stimulation* (or *e-stim*). This electrical stimulation can be useful to treat pain as is discussed in the section on TENS therapy below. The e-stim can also be useful to strengthen the pelvic floor muscles by causing muscle contractions. But how does this all relate to urinary leakage?

The muscles of the pelvic floor are important for the maintenance of our normal urinary (and, for that matter, fecal) continence. *Urinary stress incontinence* (urine leakage caused by coughing, sneezing, or laughing) is often associated with muscle weakening and poor muscle control. Building up the muscles often results in a decrease in leakage episodes and in the volume of leakage. Using complex neurological pathways, biofeedback and e-stim therapy also have been found to be useful for patients with *urinary urgency incontinence*, a form of urinary leakage caused by abnormal bladder contractions (the "overactive bladder").

Now, the big question remains: Can biofeedback and e-stim improve the symptoms of IC? The answer is yes, particularly if pelvic floor spasm is present. In carefully selected patients 69 percent had improvement in symptoms (Mendelowitz and Moldwin 1997). Biofeedback therapy has also been found to be useful in the treatment of vulvar pain syndromes (Glazer, Rodke, Swencionis, Hertz, et al. 1995).

Some Caveats About Biofeedback

1. When used for the treatment of interstitial cystitis, biofeedback and e-stim therapy should be performed only by practitioners who have special training in pelvic floor dysfunction and pain. The problem here is that *biofeedback, when applied in the same fashion for IC as for urinary incontinence, can worsen the symptoms of IC*. These procedures usually are performed by physical therapists, biofeedback specialists, doctors, or nurses.

2. Biofeedback and/or e-stim can cause a worsening of IC symptoms during the first few treatments. This problem usually settles down after the first few applications.

3. These are labor-intensive procedures. Initially, they require many sessions in the office (this varies from clinician to clinician). If the procedure is helpful, consideration usually is given to buying or leasing a home biofeedback unit.

Transcutaneous Electrical Nerve Stimulation (TENS) Therapy

TENS therapy has been used for the treatment of pain for the last twenty to thirty years. The therapy involves placing electrodes on the skin's surface. When used for home therapy, a clip-on belt stimulator unit creates a small electrical charge that runs between the electrodes and slowly desensitizes the underlying nerves. While the TENS unit is running, you will feel a tingling of the area being treated. The stimulation has been likened to "white noise" for the nerves. The nerves of the affected area become so busy processing signals about the white noise that they have difficulty transmitting pain information: essentially, the nerves are overloaded. TENS therapy also seems to stimulate the body's production of *endorphins*, the normally produced narcotic pain relievers that the body manufactures by itself.

TENS therapy can be delivered to the IC patient through electrodes attached to the lower abdomen. Alternatively, a vaginal probe with attached electrodes can be used. Most clinicians these days use the vaginal probe because the therapy can be administered as close as possible to the bladder, pelvic floor muscles, and nerves. The probe is usually the same as that used with biofeedback. Abdominal electrodes are used primarily for women who just can't tolerate any foreign body in their vaginas.

Most of the research regarding TENS therapy for interstitial cystitis comes from the studies of Fall, Carlsson, and Erlandson (1980) and Fall (1987) in Sweden. Dr. Fall and his group found surprisingly good results using this technique; but, like biofeedback, the best results were achieved with very frequent use of long duration. Sixteen of twenty patients with "classical" disease (associated with bladder scarring and severe bladder inflammation) rated the therapy as "good" to "excellent." Interestingly, patients with "nonclassical" disease (no associated scarring or significant bladder inflammation) did not fare as well.

Stress Reduction

Periodic stress is a normal part of everybody's life. Physiologically, our bodies are prepared to deal with it. However, problems seem to begin when stress becomes constant and severe as seen in many patients with IC. Multiple studies have suggested that stress can have a negative effect on our immune systems. Stress is frequently associated with recurrences of herpes and other infections, and it also has been found to incite episodes of acute asthma.

To focus on the bladder, animal studies have demonstrated that stress induces mast cells (specialized inflammatory cells, often seen in high numbers in the bladder walls of IC patients) of the bladder to release histamine, a chemical that induces inflammation (Spanos, Pang, Ligris, Letourneau, et al. 1997). Koziol, Clark, Gittes, and Tan (1993) found that stress increased symptoms in 61 percent of their IC patients.

We have found that increased levels of stress most significantly affect those patients who have spasm of the pelvic floor muscles. Those patients tend to unconsciously tighten their pelvic muscles when stress levels are climbing. Dealing with the stress is therefore just as important as any conventional medical management. Details regarding methods of stress management are well beyond the scope of this text. However, some methods that get favorable reviews from IC patients include the following:

1. **Progressive muscle relaxation.** Developed in the 1970s, this simple technique tightens, then progressively relaxes specific muscle groups. The technique is practiced with a therapist in face-to-face sessions. Stress reducing audiotapes are often used in conjunction with this therapy. At our institution, 86 percent of patients who were taught the technique used it regularly. Seventy-six percent of patients felt that it improved their urological condition. Forty-three percent noted that it helped other medical and/or psychological problems, and 93 percent would recommend relaxation training to others. This is clearly a potentially very helpful method of self-care that has absolutely no downside.

2. **Diaphragmatic breathing.** Slow diaphragmatic breathing (using your diaphragm to move air in and out of your lungs as opposed to using your rib cage) has a general calming effect on the nervous system. Diaphragmatic breathing also promotes progressive muscle relaxation.

3. **Hypnosis.** Hypnosis has been used in the management of pain with variable results. Although hypnosis has been helpful for patients in the management of stress and to facilitate muscle relaxation, we've found it to be disappointing for pain control.

4. **Yoga and tai chi.** Yoga, originally introduced to the United States in the early 1900s, has been practiced in India for centuries. Its goals are to provide mental, spiritual, and physical discipline. Various forms of yoga exist but most incorporate diaphragmatic breathing and meditation. Participants assume many poses (or *asanas*) that involve stretching and muscle strengthening. Some yoga programs incorporate some aerobic activities. Tai chi chuan (the full name for tai chi) is an ancient form of low-impact exercise and meditation that developed in China as an offshoot of the martial arts. Slow, choreographed ballet-like movements coordinated with breathing are performed to develop a harmonious flow of *chi*, or body energy. Tai chi is another excellent form of meditation. It also has a focus on progressive muscle relaxation and can improve body coordination and balance. Many community centers and local health clubs run yoga or tai chi classes. People who are new to any form of exercise might find yoga the best to begin with. But, be careful! There are forms of both disciplines that can be too strenuous for you. Many of the positions assumed by both yoga and tai chi involve deep knee bending. This, of course, can pose a problem if you have pre-existing knee troubles. The best advice is to discuss your medical condition with your instructor before you start the course. An instructor might even be able to incorporate some techniques to promote relaxation of the pelvic muscles.

5. **Massage therapy.** Therapeutic massage can reduce stress and may also be useful in pain management. Just as with yoga and tai chi, many techniques of massage are based upon Asian principles of body energy flow. Usually registered massage therapists or physical therapists administer massage. Before you start therapy, make sure that you discuss your medical problem with your therapist. He or she might decide to use one form of massage over another based upon what you tell them.

6. **The role of mental health workers.** Chronic stress is frequently associated with panic attacks and depression. It's

always important to share these issues with your doctor; however, sometimes their "office flow" precludes serious counseling. Furthermore, most medical specialists (urologists, gynecologists, etc.) haven't been trained to manage these problems effectively. Psychologists and psychiatric social workers can help a great deal with these issues. Don't be afraid to contact them if needed. Sometimes, a psychiatrist's skills may be needed, particularly when medications for depression or severe anxiety are needed.

7. **The role of other IC patients.** IC patients share numerous common problems. Discussing these issues in a support group setting has the advantage of making one feel less alone. It's often helpful to hear the various coping strategies that other people use. Perhaps you can incorporate them into your own life. Helping other people in the same boat can be therapeutic all by itself. By far, the best group to become involved with is the Interstitial Cystitis Association (ICA), 51 Monroe Street, Suite 1402, Rockville, MD 20850, (301) 610-5300 or www.ichelp.org. Articles and books that cover topics like psychological, sexual, and relationship issues as well as treatment options, disability issues, and self-help strategies are available through the ICA's Resource Materials Guide.

Protocols for Bladder Retraining

The typical interstitial cystitis patient urinates small volumes on a frequent basis because of pelvic discomfort or urinary urgency. That sense of needing to find the bathroom is caused by bladder oversensitivity, and doesn't always coincide with the bladder's true capacity. Unfortunately, by going to the bathroom very often, the bladder never has a chance to stretch and maintain its size. Rather, the bladder often slowly shrinks since it is rarely completely filled. This creates a vicious cycle where the slow decrease in bladder size makes you want to go to the bathroom even more frequently; the bladder then fills to a smaller volume and thereby shrinks some more.

Many of the therapies that help the IC patient work by decreasing the bladder's sensitivity. If the bladder is not as sensitive, it can fill more effectively. Another way to deal with the problem is to slowly *retrain* the bladder to hold more fluid. Bladder retraining seems to help increase the size (capacity) of the bladder and, in some patients, it decreases the bladder's sensitivity.

The goal of bladder retraining therapy is to *slowly* increase the duration between voids. The key to the process is to keep a diary of the times that you urinate. The average time between voids is noted and serves as a baseline. The next step is to try and hold your urine perhaps ten to fifteen minutes longer. This might be continued for a week. Then, the interval between voids can be increased further and further as the weeks go by. The progression is very much determined by the patient and the severity of their disease.

Another approach to increasing your bladder's size is to always try holding off urination ten to twenty minutes after you feel the need to urinate. Over time, many patients note that the overall duration between voids progressively increases. This slightly different approach to bladder retraining should be monitored by your caregiver. Fifty to seventy percent of patients will have "significant" symptom improvement using a bladder retraining protocol. Within twelve weeks, some patients are able to increase their voiding intervals from one hour to three hours. Note that patients who experience a great deal of associated pain are not good candidates for this approach.

Key Points About Bladder Retraining

1. It can take a long time to see results, often up to three months. Patients who have very small and scarred bladders may need to continue this protocol for six to twelve months to see any improvement.

2. Many patients note that the protocol allows them to hold more urine, but the sensation to urinate still comes on pretty early. This is probably the biggest complaint from our patients. If a decrease in pelvic discomfort is to occur, it comes toward the end of therapy (three months), so it's important to hang in there!

3. There is no question that a bladder retraining protocol is best done under the supervision of trained medical personnel, usually a medical social worker or a nurse clinician. They are able to keep you on track and make adjustments in the voiding intervals as needed.

4. Bladder retraining appears to have the best results when done in combination with other therapies such as biofeedback or stress management.

5. Pain must be controlled prior to proceeding with bladder retraining.

Physical Therapy

Physical therapy can be extremely helpful to the IC patient, particularly for those patients who have associated spasm of the pelvic floor muscles. Many physical therapists have received training to deal specifically with pelvic pain syndromes. Some have even made it their area of specialization. Their services may include biofeedback, e-stim, therapeutic massage, relaxation training, exercise programming, and myofascial release (manual stretching of spastic, sensitive muscles and associated structures). Myofascial release of the pelvic floor muscles is often performed through the vagina in women and through the rectum in men. If you or your caregiver is interested in finding a physical therapist specializing in this area, your best bet is to call the American Physical Therapists Association at 800-999-2782, extension 3387.

Acupuncture

Acupuncture is one of the oldest medical therapies, dating back over 5,000 years. It is based upon the belief that our health is maintained through a balanced flow of body energy. This energy is thought to proceed through twelve channels called meridians and approximately 1,000 acupoints. Disruptions in the energy flow can result in disease or pain. Acupuncture technique involves inserting needles (sometimes spinning the needles or introducing electricity through them) into specific acupoints, depending on the condition that needs to be treated, to "rebalance" the flow of energy. It's thought by some that acupuncture works much the same way as TENS (see the section on TENS therapy earlier in this chapter). Acupressure, a variant of acupuncture, uses pressure rather than the insertion of needles.

Current literature suggests that acupuncture can improve pelvic pain and symptoms of urinary urgency and frequency. However, there are few well-performed studies. Acupuncture appears to be particularly useful for the treatment of menstrual pain. In 1987, Helms demonstrated that "real" acupuncture resulted in 90.9 percent of patients with less pelvic pain, where only 36 percent of patients given placebo acupuncture (the needles in this group were purposely placed incorrectly) reported symptom improvement. Most importantly, the real acupuncture group had a 41 percent reduction in their use of analgesic medication.

To date, few studies have evaluated the role of acupuncture for the interstitial cystitis patient. One study by Geirsson, Wang, Lindstrom, and Fall (1993) didn't demonstrate any significant change in IC symptoms after therapy. The symptom reduction was short-lived in the one patient who had a favorable response to therapy.

Our impression of acupuncture in the treatment of pelvic pain is that if it is to work, just as with TENS therapy, it takes time—at least two months of weekly to biweekly sessions. Acupuncture also seems to be operator-dependent. There are people who perform acupuncture quite well and achieve reasonable results, and, of course, there are those practitioners who hardly ever get good results. Because we've seen the results of acupuncture to be far from impressive, we usually don't recommend this as early therapy. Before you get started with an acupuncturist, make sure to ask him or her if they've had any experiences dealing with pelvic pain, and with bladder problems in particular. One of the best sources of information can be other patients whom you meet on the Internet, at ICA (Interstitial Cystitis Association) support meetings, or through phone conversations with local ICA support staff.

The Role of Vitamin Therapy

Vitamins and minerals are chemicals normally found in our food that are essential for carrying out the basic metabolic functions of our bodies. Certain vitamins and minerals have been shown to participate in nerve function, blood flow, wound healing, and the immune system—processes that are especially important to the IC patient. You should be able to get all the vitamins and minerals that you need from your diet. Unfortunately, the diet of many IC patients is far from ideal due to multiple food sensitivities. It, therefore, may pay to take a daily multivitamin supplement. *There is no scientific evidence to support improvement in the symptoms of IC using any specific vitamin/mineral regime.* Specific vitamins and minerals that are *probably* most important for the IC patient include the following:

Vitamin A (Retinol)

Vitamin A is a fat-soluble compound that serves an important role in our immune and nervous systems. Vitamin A deficiency can result in night blindness, color vision abnormalities, poor coordination, a loss of taste, smell, and appetite. Most people get plenty of vitamin A in their diets as vitamin A's precursor, beta-carotene. One needs to be cautious with vitamin A supplementation since toxic levels can result in liver disease. If you are pregnant, be especially careful about vitamin A supplementation since even the dosages found in some multivitamins have been associated with miscarriages and birth defects.

Food sources: Tuna fish, carrots, pumpkin, butternut squash, spinach, sweet potatoes, turnip greens, mangoes. (Note that the lists of foods supplied in this section may be on the "no-no" list for IC patients. Please remember that not all foods on that list will affect every IC patient. It's important to experiment with your diet!)

Daily recommended intake: 5,000 International Units (IU)

Vitamin B6 (Pyridoxine)

Vitamin B6 plays an important role in our nervous systems. Vitamin B6 deficiency is known to lead to nerve damage, memory loss, and glucose intolerance. Overdosage is associated with skin sensitivity to sunlight and nerve disorders. Vitamin B6 supplements may interfere with therapy for Parkinson's disease, so consult your doctor.

Food sources: Oats, whole wheat, eggs, chicken, fish, beef, brewer's yeast, brown rice, peanuts, soybeans, walnuts, bananas, avocados

Daily recommended intake: 2 milligrams (mg)

Vitamin C (Ascorbic Acid)

Vitamin C is an antioxidant that has multiple beneficial effects on the body. It seems to be important in the normal maintenance of our immune and cardiovascular systems. It also has an important role in wound healing, being intimately involved with collagen production. Some IC patients have complained of worsening symptoms with vitamin C supplementation. Buffered preparations reportedly cause fewer problems. Vitamin C deficiency can lead to lethargy and delayed wound healing. In its most severe form, vitamin C deficiency can lead to scurvy whose symptoms include muscle weakness and pain, bleeding gums, and mental status changes

Food sources: Oranges, cantaloupe, peppers, grapefruit, kiwis, strawberries, pineapple, kidney, liver, fish

Daily recommended intake: 60 mg (higher doses of 100–1,000 mg have been recommended for smokers or in postoperative patients)

Vitamin E (D-alpha tocopherol)

Vitamin E is another antioxidant that plays an important role in our immune, nervous, and cardiovascular systems. Vitamin E can lower the body's level of histamine, a potential benefit for the IC patient. Vitamin E deficiency is rare. People who take anticoagulants (blood thinners) should not take vitamin E supplements due to the possibility of excessive bleeding. As well, you should consult with your doctor if you have a history of stroke or bleeding tendencies.

Food sources: Whole grains, vegetable and nut oils, sunflower seeds, wheat germ, spinach

Daily recommended intake: 30 IU

Zinc

Zinc is an important mineral for our immune and nervous systems. Free zinc has a well-established role as an antibacterial agent in the prostate gland. Zinc is also essential for wound healing. We should get most of the zinc that we need from our diet. Unfortunately, the low fat diet many people follow these days excludes red meats and eggs, two excellent sources of zinc. Signs of zinc deficiency include fatigue, loss of taste and smell, night blindness, skin rashes, hair loss, changes in the menstrual cycle, and depression.

Food sources: Red meat, lamb, eggs, whole grains, oysters, yogurt, nuts

Daily recommended intake: 15 mg

Calcium

Calcium is an important mineral that participates in multiple cellular activities and is an essential component to muscle and nerve function. Calcium supplementation has received much attention in the lay and medical press due to the high incidence of osteoporosis seen in postmenopausal women. Calcium requirements vary from person to person, based upon their age, sex, menstrual or pregnancy status. The daily calcium needs are generally highest with adolescence (1,200 to 1,500 mg), menopause (1,500 mg) (without estrogen replacement), pregnancy (1,200 mg). and after sixty-five years of age (1,500 mg). Too much calcium can lead to constipation, and will inhibit zinc and iron absorption. Many IC patients use antacids for calcium supplementation (calcium carbonate). Make sure to use aluminum-free calcium (like TUMS or Rolaids) if you choose any form of calcium supplement, since aluminum prevents bone mineralization.

Food sources: Cheeses, skim milk, collard greens, broccoli, canned salmon or sardines with bones, corn tortillas processed with lime, mustard greens
Daily recommended intake: See above

Manganese

Manganese works along with calcium to maintain strong bones and connective tissue. It is also important to the normal function of our nervous system. Excessive doses of calcium can prevent manganese absorption. To compensate for calcium supplementation, eating foods rich in manganese later in the day is recommended.
Food sources: Canned pineapple juice, wheat bran, wheat germ, whole grains, nuts, shellfish, tea
Daily recommended intake: 2 mg

Please note that the daily recommended intakes listed above represent those established by the Food and Drug Administration. As mentioned earlier, there is no current evidence that taking high doses of any vitamin or mineral will relieve the symptoms of IC. However, if you are interested in proceeding with therapy beyond a daily multivitamin, it would probably be best to do this under the guidance of a nutritionist or a clinician experienced in this area.
Other good sources of information include the following:

* The *USP Guide to Vitamins and Minerals.* Call HarperCollins at 800-331-3761.

* *Consumer Reports on Health*, "Vitamins and Minerals, and Herbs—Oh My! (When it comes to the selling of dietary supplements, it's a jungle out there. We'll guide you through.)" April 1998, vol. 10, no. 4, pp. 6-8.

* *Consumer Reports on Health*, "Smart About Supplements? (Test yourself with our not-so-easy questions about vitamins, herbs, and other dietary supplements.)" February 2000, vol. 12, no. 2, pp. 7-10.

Herbs

As little as can be said about vitamins and their role in IC, less can be said about phytotherapy (the clinical use of herbs). Nevertheless, patients are spending lots of money on some of these remedies. Fortunately, the National Institutes of Health has recently opened a new office of Alternative and Complementary Medicine. We are all anxiously waiting to see the true effects of these therapies when placed under standard scientific scrutiny. The most popular herbal therapies for IC (at least what most people are finding during chat sessions on the Internet) include aloe vera, marshmallow root, spirulina (blue-green algae), and chondroitin sulfate (see chapter 5, Oral Therapies for IC). These therapies supposedly improve the quality of the bladder lining; however, apart from anecdotes, we are unaware of any scientific evidence to support these claims.

The bioflavonoid, quercetin, was recently evaluated for the treatment of male chronic pelvic pain syndrome, Type III A and B (in some instances, this problem has been associated with IC. See chapter 7, The Male with Interstitial Cystitis) (Shoskes, Zeitlin, Shahed, and Rajfer 1999). Quercetin appears to inhibit histamine release from mast cells. Using a dose of 500 mg, twice daily for one month, they demonstrated that 67 percent of patients had at least a 25 percent decrease in their symptoms while only 20 percent of patients taking placebo had this response.

Chapter **11**

Support for the Interstitial Cystitis Patient

By Vicki Ratner, M.D. (ICA Founder and President)

Pain Without Respite

For much of the twentieth century, interstitial cystitis (IC) was over-looked, misunderstood, and misdiagnosed by the medical commu-nity. People with IC were sometimes forced to live a lifetime with intractable physical pain, compounded by the emotional pain of being told that nothing was wrong, or even being blamed for their condition. Although attitudes by the medical community are chang-ing today, there are still physicians who don't believe that IC is real. The ICA (Interstitial Cystitis Association) often receives letters from patients who do not receive adequate treatment. One woman wrote, "Sometimes I wish I were dead because the misery and pain are unbearable. If I had cancer, I would know sooner or later that I would be either in remission or dead, but with IC, I suffer day after day, without any hope of getting better. So many times I have thought of killing myself to get out of the pain and mental suffering caused by this disease." Another patient wrote, "I have constant, intense, unrelenting, deep pain and hard as I try, mentally, physi-cally, and emotionally, I cannot stand it for long without relief. I feel like I'm being tortured without respite" (Ratner and Slade 1997). Chronic pain can lead to depression and thoughts of suicide, testi-mony to the truth of Dr. Albert Schweitzer's statement: "Pain is a more terrible lord of mankind than even death itself."

The lack of medical knowledge about IC is not surprising, since no federal funding was available for research on IC, its epidemiology, diagnosis, treatment, and its possible cause(s), until 1987. This funding and renewed interest was prompted by the work of the Interstitial Cystitis Association (ICA), founded in 1984. Today, new research has begun to shed light on all aspects of this long neglected disorder.

The Doctor Becomes a Patient

I was a third-year medical student when my IC symptoms began. I had just delivered my first baby while on my obstetrics and gynecology rotation. But pain overshadowed the excitement of my very first delivery. Thinking it was just another of many urinary tract infections, I started drinking lots of water, dropped off a urine specimen at the lab, and began taking antibiotics. But the steady discomfort quickly changed to sharp, persistent pain. Urine cultures proved negative, antibiotics didn't help, and more tests showed nothing. I received no relief from the pain for the next eighteen months. It was 1984 and I was thirty-four years old.

The pain was relentless and debilitating, like having a permanent urinary tract infection. After visits to ten urologists, two allergists, and two infectious disease specialists, I was sent home with a diagnosis of stress, a referral to a psychiatrist, and a recommendation to quit medical school and get married. Instead, I went to the library. There I read about a disease called interstitial cystitis. The book's description of IC spoke volumes about physicians' prevailing negative attitudes toward women.

So I wasn't surprised that my original urologist disagreed with the diagnosis of IC, saying that I was too young. When I insisted, my urologist reluctantly performed a cystoscopy under general anesthesia and the diagnosis of IC was finally confirmed. Interstitial cystitis was also included in the psychosomatic disorders chapter in *Campbell's Urology*, the standard urology textbook used in the United States. This is the information that I found, as I was desperately seeking answers: [IC is] "a disease that . . . may represent the end stage of a bladder that has been made irritable by emotional disturbance. . . . A pathway for the discharge of unconscious hatreds" (*Campbell's Urology* 1979).

Naming the condition validated my judgment and assured me that I wasn't crazy, but finding a treatment that worked proved incredibly difficult. I spent the last two years of medical school in intense, unremitting pain and isolation. I thought I was the only one in the world with this disease.

The Politics of Disease

This painful experience taught me many lessons that changed my life and the way I practice medicine today. Two of the most important lessons: First, trust your own judgment. Second, medical problems sometimes have political solutions. AIDS and breast cancer are two perfect examples. When patients speak up and speak out, demanding public attention and research funding for their disease, they make a difference.

My library research showed me how little was known about the treatment of IC and how little interest there was in learning more. Initial appeals to the National Institutes of Health (NIH)—the medical research arm of the U.S. government, the Centers for Disease Control (CDC), and the American Urologic Association (AUA) produced no results. So in 1985, as a last resort, I talked with a local reporter about IC and that led to a three-minute appearance on the ABC network program, "Good Morning, America."

Within one week of that appearance, ten thousand letters poured in from women who had endured the physical pain of IC for years as well as the emotional pain of physicians' dismissal and denial. Their stories echoed my own experience: all of these women had gone from doctor to doctor to doctor, looking for relief from severe pain and frequent urination, despite negative urine cultures. From this outpouring of anguish, I saw the elements of an advocacy organization that could make a difference for people who suffered from interstitial cystitis.

Together with a small group of other IC patients, I founded the Interstitial Cystitis Association (ICA), which has become the primary mechanism for improving education, awareness, and research funding for interstitial cystitis.

Patient Advocacy Changes Everything

The Interstitial Cystitis Association that began in my New York City living room in 1984 bears little resemblance to the organization today. Now the leading national nonprofit organization for IC, the ICA is headquartered in Rockville, Maryland, just outside of Washington, D.C. Growing an advocacy organization took time, money, and a team of dedicated staff and volunteers working together toward a common goal. Working together taught us that medical issues are political issues and it became clear that help for people with IC would take advocacy, education, support, and research. Those elements became the cornerstones of the ICA.

The history of the ICA is the story of continued effort and steady progress. Until 1987, no federal research money had been spent on interstitial cystitis, but relentless advocacy by the ICA changed that. Many meetings with policy makers on Capitol Hill and testimony at Congressional hearings led to the first Congressional appropriation of federal funds for IC research at NIH. Continuing support from NIH and Congress has helped to develop a research community interested in this disease.

While continuing to encourage the NIH to become involved in IC research, the ICA simultaneously sought research funding to establish its own Pilot Research Program. What makes the ICA unique is that it provides and administers funding opportunities for IC research in the U.S. and around the world. Currently, the ICA offers interested IC researchers two programs. The ICA's Pilot Research Program provides initial support, or "seed money," to help researchers gather preliminary data before applying for funding from the NIH or larger private foundations. In addition, the ICA also administers the Fishbein Family IC Research Foundation Grant Program.

Establishing a nationwide support network for IC patients was of utmost importance to the ICA. This large support network is described in the following section as are the ICA educational publications and programs for both patients and physicians. This educational effort continues to be important in overcoming the paucity of information available about IC.

Where to Turn for Support

When confronted with the symptoms of a debilitating, poorly understood, chronic illness such as IC, it is easy to feel extremely isolated. You may have suffered with symptoms of the disease for years, going from doctor to doctor trying to get a correct diagnosis. Once diagnosed, you face a trial-and-error period of treatment possibilities. Because the cause or causes of IC remain unknown, many of the questions you may have about IC are unanswerable.

Interstitial cystitis can disrupt every aspect of your life. Severe pain, sleep deprivation, and frequent trips to the bathroom can make it difficult to maintain relationships with your spouse or significant other, family, and friends, as well as adding difficulties with holding a job or participating in daily social activities.

Support services can make a critical difference in coping with IC and more of these services are available than ever before. From support groups, web site and Internet connections, to publications for patients, telephone support, regional and national educational meetings, and disability services, the array of services is quite extensive.

Publications for Interstitial Cystitis Patients

Most IC patients find that keeping abreast of current information helps them to cope better with their illness. The ICA publishes the *ICA Update*, a quarterly newsletter that provides comprehensive, up-to-date information about IC treatments, self-help strategies, research, and clinical trials. It also provides current information on new medications being tested by the FDA, summaries of the latest research studies, and updates on federal funding from Congress. Each issue of the *ICA Update* includes the ICA Resource Materials Guide, which details available resources such as articles reprinted from medical journals, transcripts of ICA regional and national conferences, booklets on disability, and numerous fact sheets and brochures. In addition, the ICA publishes *Visions*, a quarterly newsletter for ICA volunteers. The National Institute of Diabetes, Digestive and Kidney Diseases (NIDDK) also publishes a free booklet for IC patients. You can order a copy of this publication by contacting the National Kidney and Urologic Diseases Information Clearinghouse (NKUDIC) at 3 Information Way, Bethesda, MD 20892-3580. To view this publication online, go to http://www.niddk.nih.gov/health/kidney/kidney.htm

Local Support Groups

Currently, the ICA has a dedicated volunteer network of 200 people from across the country. Many of these volunteers take on a leadership role as Support Group Leaders and oversee the planning and facilitating of local support group meetings. There are also IC-related support groups that are not affiliated with the ICA.

Some patients choose support groups that address more general needs such as coping with chronic illness or pain. Others choose support groups that address chronic conditions associated with IC, such as fibromyalgia or Sjogren's syndrome.

Telephone Support

Part of the ICA volunteer network includes national ICA Telephone Support Volunteers. These knowledgeable volunteers return calls promptly and offer suggestions and encouragement to IC patients. The ICA also offers the Phone Friends program, which gives IC patients an additional opportunity to support and encourage each other. Specialized phone support is available for men with IC, patients contemplating surgery, patients with Hunner's ulcers, patients considering pregnancy, and patients with related conditions such as fibromyalgia and vulvodynia. Additional support is made available for more complex IC-related questions through the ICA by calling 1-800-HELP-ICA.

Regional and National Educational Meetings

The ICA sponsors a biannual national meeting for patients, caregivers, researchers, and clinicians to meet and exchange information. In conjunction with each national meeting, the ICA cosponsors with the NIDDK a scientific symposium where researchers from all over the world present their most current research findings. The ICA also sponsors IC Regional Forums throughout the country, featuring leading IC experts who present the most up-to-date information about interstitial cystitis.

Internet Support

The advent of the Internet has brought about dramatic changes in the way information is obtained. Web sites, chat rooms, message boards, and e-mail lists are now available. The ICA offers a comprehensive web site located at www.ichelp.org, which brings together the latest research news and educational information for patients and physicians. The ICA's web site also provides a place for patients to ask questions about concerns regarding their condition. Over 500,000 visits to the ICA web site are made every month by patients from all over the world.

The Interstitial Cystitis Network, a for-profit medical publishing company, provides a web site with message boards, chat rooms, and weekly presentations on IC (see the Resources section).The Urologychannel.com, which is also a commercial web site, makes information on IC available and has a message board where patients' questions are posted along with urologists' responses. Mediconsult (www.mediconsult.com) is a medical health care site that also provides comprehensive information on IC as well as a message board. For America Online (AOL) users, AOL offers a highly frequented IC message board and weekly chat rooms. Please contact the ICA to find out the location of the AOL IC message board.

Finding an IC-Knowledgeable Physician

The ICA publishes a fact sheet entitled *Finding the Right Physician for You* which many patients find helpful. Another useful resource is *A Delicate Balance: Living Successfully with Chronic Illness* (1998) by IC patient and writer Susan Milstrey Wells. This is an excellent self-help book that also has an informative section on how to choose a doctor. The ICA distributes, upon request, the Physician Registry, a state-by-state list of urologists who have indicated their interest in treating patients with IC. The Interstital Cystitis Network also lists physicians interested in IC on their web site. Interstitial cystitis patients who are seeking help with pain management can contact one of the pain management organizations listed in the Resource section in the back of this book. Some of these organizations have pain management specialists listed by state on their web sites.

Advocacy Services

The ICA continues to advocate for funding specifically earmarked for research on the causes, epidemiology, and treatment of interstitial cystitis. These efforts extend beyond meetings on Capitol Hill to private sector corporations and pharmaceutical companies.

Disability Services

The ICA works to educate doctors about the necessity of providing support and written reports on disability for patients with severe and disabling IC. They also assist patients in preparing for and winning disability benefits from the Social Security Administration (SSA) and private insurers. The ICA provides excellent printed resource materials to assist both patients and physicians to document and win disability benefits. (Call the ICA for further assistance.)

Support for Related Conditions

Some patients with IC may experience other chronic conditions in addition to IC such as allergies, irritable bowel syndrome, fibromyalgia, migraines, lupus erythematosus, endometriosis, and vulvodynia (Alagiri, Chottiner, Ratner, Slade, et al. 1997). Researchers believe that these associations occur only in a subset of IC patients. Why these conditions are more prevalent among patients with IC is unclear, indicating the need for more research in this most important area.

For additional help on related disorders, contact the organizations listed in the Resources section at the back of the book.

Looking Ahead

The advocacy efforts of the ICA have yielded dramatic results. Fifteen years ago, the outlook for patients with IC was bleak. Interstitial cystitis was an orphan disease, misunderstood and misdiagnosed by physicians and ignored by researchers. Today, thanks to the ICA, patients are diagnosed more quickly and they have access to a wide array of treatments. The ICA's continued education of physicians and researchers has led to increased awareness, vastly increased scientific knowledge, and a willingness among many physicians to work in partnership with patients to individualize treatment regimens. The education of policy makers has led to federal funding for IC, which ensures continued research. This research has brought us close to finding a diagnostic marker for IC that will lead to more effective treatments and, ultimately, to a cure.

However, in spite of the fact that tremendous progress has been made, there are still physicians who think that IC does not exist. It still can take years for a patient to be diagnosed and properly treated. Until the cause of IC is clearly understood, and new, more effective treatments become available, relieving the symptoms of this debilitating condition must be a priority while the research continues. The continued education of physicians about IC as a treatable clinical disorder can relieve needless suffering for patients and foster collaborative efforts for finding relief for their symptoms, until a cure is found.

For more information about support services offered by the ICA, please contact:

ICA
51 Monroe St., Suite 1402
Rockville, MD 20850
Toll free: 1-800-HELP-ICA
Tel: (301) 610-5300   Fax: (301) 610-5308
E-mail: ICinfo@ichelp. org   Web site: www.IChelp.org

For additional sources of help, be sure to check out the Resources section at the back of the book.

The author wishes to gratefully acknowledge the assistance of Lucretia Perilli in the preparation of this manuscript.

Glossary

Acontractile: Having no contractions. When used in a urological sense, this term usually refers to a bladder that has no ability to contract and thereby release urine properly.

Acute: A condition of sudden onset. The opposite of acute is *chronic.* A chronic condition is long-lasting.

Acute Prostatitis (*Category I Prostatitis*): A form of prostatitis caused by bacteria, usually causing severe acute signs and symptoms such as fever, chills, burning with urination, and difficulty urinating.

Allergy: A rapid response from the body's immune system against a foreign substance. Allergies usually manifest with symptoms ranging from a runny nose and nasal congestion to hives. In its most severe form called "anaphylaxis," it may be associated with a significant drop in blood pressure, closing down of the breathing passages, and even death. Nausea, stomach upset, or fatigue associated with certain foods or medications are not typical signs of allergy.

Anesthetic: Medications that decrease the sensation of pain. Anesthetics can be broken down into several groups, as follows:

> *Topical:* Anesthetic is applied directly to a surface.

> *Local:* Anesthetic is injected into the painful site or the area surrounding it.

> *General:* The patient loses consciousness.

> *IV sedation:* Medications are administered through an intravenous line. These medications cause the patient to become very relaxed or they can be administered to the point where the patient falls into a deep sleep. All the while, the patient is

breathing normally. Therefore, as a rule, no anesthetic mask or breathing tube placement is needed.

Spinal: The anesthetizing agent is injected into the space surrounding the lower portion of the spinal cord. This produces the inability to move or to sense pain or touch in the lower portion of the body.

Epidural: This also involves placing a needle into the region surrounding the spinal cord. The needle does not penetrate as deeply as it does for spinal anesthesia. Additionally, a very skinny tube (catheter) is left in place of the epidural needle. The catheter transports anesthetic medications to the nerves exiting the spine, thus providing excellent pain control. The epidural catheter can be left in place for long periods of time, thus providing the patient with a duration of pain control that can far exceed that achieved with spinal anesthesia.

Antibiotics: Medications commonly used to treat bacterial infections. Most antibiotics do not have any effect on fungal or viral infections.

Anticholinergic Medications: These medications cause relaxation of the muscles within the bladder. This group of medications may also affect the muscle within the intestines, sometimes causing constipation. They are also well-known to cause dryness of the mouth because of their ability to decrease saliva production.

Antioxidant: A chemical that has the ability to neutralize molecules called "free radicals." *Free radicals* are unstable chemicals that can cause tissue damage. Their damage to DNA molecules has been implicated in the development of cancer.

Antiseptic: A medication that kills microorganisms on contact. These medications, when taken orally, usually achieve high concentrations in the urine; however, as a rule, they have very poor tissue penetration. They are, therefore, excellent medications for superficial urinary tract infections, but are not that helpful in the treatment of deep-seated infections.

Asymptomatic: Having no symptoms.

Asymptomatic Bacteriuria: Bacteria found in the urine; however, there are no accompanying symptoms of a urinary tract infection such as urinary urgency, frequency, or burning.

Atrophic Vaginitis: A condition in which the lining of the vagina looses thickness and becomes thin and dry. This usually is caused by a loss of estrogen and can result in symptoms of vaginal itching and/or burning, loss of vaginal lubrication, and discomfort with sexual intercourse.

Autoimmune Disease: A condition where the body is attacked by its own immune system.

Benign Prostatic Hyperplasia (BPH): The normal growth of the prostate as the male ages. In some cases, this growth may cause obstruction to the flow of urine.

Biopsy: To take a small sample of tissue for analysis.

Biofeedback: The technique of making unconscious or involuntary bodily processes (such as the activity of your pelvic floor muscles) perceptible to the senses (as is often demonstrated on a computer screen) in order to manipulate them by conscious mental control.

Bladder Neck: The region at the base of the bladder where urine exits into the urethra.

Bladder Capacity: How much fluid the bladder can hold. The bladder capacity usually refers to the amount of fluid that can be held while you're awake. The *anesthetic bladder capacity* refers to the amount that can be held while the patient is under anesthesia.

Bladder Surface Mucin: A thin "protective" lining of the bladder surface. Its two apparent main functions are: 1. To prevent bacteria from adhering to the bladder surface, and 2. To protect the bladder surface from noxious chemicals present in the urine.

Catheter: A small tube usually used to drain fluid. These tubes come in varying sizes denoted by the term "French." The higher the French size, the larger the diameter of the catheter. Most catheters used for adults range from 14 to 24 French. Typically, three types of catheters are used to drain urine from the bladder:

1. *Straight catheter*: This is sometimes also called the red rubber catheter. This is simply a straight tube that is usually inserted into the urethra to drain urine. The straight catheter is only meant to drain urine and then to be removed.

2. *Foley catheter*: Very similar to the straight catheter except this is designed to be left in place. A very small port is located at the draining end of the catheter. Sterile water is infused through this port and a balloon at the tip of the catheter then fills with this fluid. The balloon inflated at the tip of the bladder prevents the catheter from falling out of the patient.

3. *Suprapubic catheter*: The suprapubic catheter is a specially designed tube that is inserted, usually under local anesthesia, to drain urine directly out of the bladder through a small opening above the pubic bone.

Chronic Bacterial Prostatitis (*Prostatitis Category II*): A smoldering infection of the prostate gland caused by bacteria and typified by recurrent urinary tract infections, discomfort between the scrotum and anus (perineum), lower back pain, and testicular pain.

Connective Tissue: As the name implies, this tissue connects together various structures of the body together. Connective tissue is found in great abundance within the skin and muscles. It is primarily composed of protein, collagen, and cells called fibroblasts.

Cystectomy: A surgical procedure to remove the bladder.

Cystitis: This is a general term for inflammation of the bladder. More specific terms to define this inflammation include the following:

> *Bacterial cystitis:* Inflammation caused by bacteria.

> *Chemical cystitis:* Inflammation caused by chemicals that might be introduced into the bladder.

> *Hemorrhagic cystitis:* Inflammation of the bladder severe enough to cause gross bleeding of the bladder wall.

> *Radiation cystitis:* Inflammation of the bladder produced by radiation therapy.

> *Eosinophilic cystitis:* A bladder disease similar to interstitial cystitis. Unlike interstitial cystitis, biopsy of the bladder wall always demonstrates inflammatory cells called "eosinophils."

Cystocoele: A "dropped bladder." The bladder, in this instance, protrudes into the vagina. (See figure 5 in chapter 2.)

Cystometrogram: A test of bladder function usually performed by instilling water or gas into the bladder through a small catheter.

Cystoscope: An instrument used to look inside the bladder. Both rigid and flexible cystoscopes are available. A rigid cystoscope is a metal instrument. The majority of urological procedures are performed through rigid cystoscopy. A flexible cystoscope usually has a smaller diameter. The tip of the flexible cystoscope bends in different directions to allow visualization of the bladder wall. This type of cystoscope is usually used for diagnostic purposes; however, some procedures can be performed with this instrument as well.

Degranulation: In this book, degranulation refers to mast cells releasing their "packets" (granules) of inflammation-causing chemicals.

Detrusor: The muscle of the bladder. Usually used synonymously with the "bladder."

Dysuria: Urethral pain (usually burning) during urination.

Endometriosis: A condition where endometrium (the lining of the uterus) is found in other parts of the body. This tissue has the ability to bleed just as uterine tissue does during the menstrual cycle.

Symptoms of endometriosis vary depending upon the location of the "implants." One to two percent of endometriosis patients will have endometrial implants on the bladder. This can give rise to complaints of pelvic pain, urinary urgency, and frequency.

Endoscopy: The examination of internal bodily structures with the aid of special instruments called endoscopes. Cytoscopy and laparoscopy are forms of endoscopy.

Endoscopic Surgery: Surgical procedures performed during endoscopy.

Epidemiology: The study of the source(s), prevalence, and distribution of disease within a given population.

Estrogen: The hormone responsible for many female sex characteristics such as breast development, the menstrual cycle, and maintenance of the vaginal lining. This hormone is also produced in men and in some plants.

Fibromyalgia: A syndrome defined by specific points of tenderness along the muscles and joints of the body.

Fulguration: The burning of tissue. Fulguration usually is used to stop bleeding but it also can be used to destroy unwanted tissue.

Glomerulations: Small bleeding points on the bladder's surface. Often seen during hydrodistention of the IC patient.

Hematuria: The presence of blood in the urine. *Gross hematuria* denotes blood in the urine that can be seen without magnification. *Microscopic hematuria* means that the blood in the urine is not visible and can be seen only with the aid of a microscope.

Histamine: A chemical released from mast cells (specialized inflammatory cells) that stimulates inflammation.

Histology: Microscopic study of the body's tissues.

Hunner's Ulcer: (Also called a Hunner's patch.) A reddened region on the bladder surface that is due to intense inflammation. This can be seen during a routine cystoscopic examination.

Hydrodistention of the Bladder: A procedure used to help establish a diagnosis of interstitial cystitis. Hydrodistention involves instilling fluid at relatively high pressure into the bladder while the patient is anesthetized.

Hypersensitivity: Heightened sensitivity of a nerve to a given stimulus. The bladder surface of the IC patient is thought to be hypersensitive, thus the feeling of fullness and discomfort occurs with only small amounts of collected urine.

Hypotension: A significant decrease in blood pressure.

Hypoxia: The lack of oxygen delivered to tissues. This may result in tissue death or abnormal functioning of the tissue.

Ileal conduit: A short segment of intestine (ileum) used to drain urine outside of the body. The ureters are connected to this piece of ileum. One end of the ileum is sewn closed. The other opening is connected to the skin. Urine drains into the ileum from the ureters. It then flows out of the body through this conduit, draining into an external urine collection bag. (See figure 11B in chapter 8.)

Incontinence (Urinary): The unwanted leakage of urine.

Intermittent Catheterization: A technique where the bladder is emptied by urethral catheterization many times per day. Catheterization usually is performed by the patient and is often called "self-intermittent catheterization (SIC)." Generally, SIC is performed by patients who don't empty their bladders well.

Internal Urinary Pouch: The creation of an internal urinary pouch is usually performed in conjunction with bladder removal. A segment of intestine is used to create a new reservoir to store urine. This newly created pouch is periodically emptied during the day (with the use of intermittent catheterization) through another segment of intestine that connects the pouch to the skin. (See figure 11C in chapter 8.)

Intravenous Pyelogram (IVP): An x-ray test of the urinary system performed by introducing a contrast medication into the bloodstream. The contrast is concentrated in the kidneys and allows the urinary tract to be seen on standard x-ray film.

Intravesical [*Intra* (inside)- *vesical* (bladder)]: Inside the bladder. Intravesical therapy usually refers to medications introduced into the bladder, usually using a catheter.

Iontophoresis: When used medically, iontophoresis refers to electrical energy enhancing the transport of a medication into a tissue.

Laparoscopy: A surgical procedure in which a telescope (laparoscope) is inserted into the abdominal cavity through a small incision. In this way the abdominal cavity can be examined. *Laparoscopic surgery* can be performed by inserting specially designed instruments through other small incisions.

Mast Cell: An inflammatory cell that contains "packets" of chemicals that stimulate inflammation such as *prostaglandins*, *histamine* and *leukotrienes*.

Mucosa: The thin lining of many body surfaces that secretes a protective, slimy substance called mucin. When referring to the bladder, the mucosa is the thin inner lining that comes in contact with urine and is protected by *bladder surface mucin*. The bladder mucosa also is called the *urothelium*.

Neurostimulation or Neuromodulation: A technique where nerves are electrically stimulated. This procedure has been found to be useful in the management of many pain syndromes. Neuromodulation also has recently been used urologically to treat bladders that function abnormally.

Nonbacterial Prostatitis (*Male Chronic Pelvic Pain Syndrome, Category IIIA*): Inflammation of the prostate without any obvious bacterial infection.

Pelvic Floor: A "hammock" of muscle and connective tissue that sits at the base of the pelvis and supports the pelvic organs. The pelvic floor has numerous functions related to defecation, urination, and sexual intercourse.

Pelvic Floor Dysfunction: Abnormal function (spasm) of the muscles comprising the pelvic floor. This is frequently associated with complaints of lower back pain, constipation, poor urinary flow, pain with sexual intercourse, or generalized pelvic pain.

Perineum: The region between the scrotum and anus or the vagina and anus.

pH (potential for hydrogen): A measurement of the acidity or alkalinity of a solution. The lower the pH, the more acidic the solution. The higher the pH, the more alkaline the solution. A pH of 7 is neither alkaline nor acidic (it is *neutral*).

Placebo: A medication or other therapy given to the patient that has no efficacy for treating any disease process. Interestingly, many patients have a favorable response to this "sugar pill." This favorable response is called the *placebo effect*. All drug evaluations are performed by separating patients into at least two groups. One group takes the actual medication and the other receives the placebo. The difference in response rates between the two groups helps determine true drug efficacy. During these studies, both groups are *blinded* (patients don't know which medications they are receiving). Many studies are *double-blinded*, meaning that neither the patients nor the investigators know who is receiving which medication until a special code is broken at the end of the study.

Postvoid Residual (PVR): The amount of urine that remains in the bladder after urination.

Prostate: A gland that resides at the neck of the bladder. Urine passes through the prostate in a region called the prostatic urethra. The role of the prostate is not completely understood. It appears to serve a role in the production of semen and also may serve some function in the prevention of urinary tract infections.

Prostatitis: Inflammation of the prostate. Prostatitis may be caused by infection. However, it is much more commonly unrelated to any obvious infection.

Prostatodynia (*Male Chronic Pelvic Pain Syndrome, Category IIIB*): The literal translation is "prostate pain"; however, in this instance, the pain, which mimics prostatitis, is actually caused by spasm of the pelvic floor muscles.

Potassium Sensitivity Test: A test to help establish a diagnosis of interstitial cystitis. The test is performed by determining if the patient is sensitive (has increased pain) to a solution of potassium chloride instilled into the bladder.

Pus: Fluid that is composed primarily of inflammatory cells (white blood cells).

Pyuria: The finding of pus (white blood cells) in the urine.

Rectocoele: The protrusion of the rectum into the vagina.

Recurrent Urinary Tract Infection: Urinary tract infections that occur more than two to three times per year.

Reflux: Reflux, in a urological sense, usually means the abnormal passage of urine from the bladder up into the ureters and potentially to the kidneys. The specific terminology generally used is *vesico* (bladder)-*uretero* (ureter) reflux. The normal urine flow goes only in one direction—from the kidney down to the bladder.

Renal: A medical term referring to the kidneys.

Resect: To remove a piece of tissue.

Seminal Vesicles: Two small glands that sit behind the bladder and connect to the prostate gland. The seminal vesicles are responsible for creating most of the fluid found in semen.

Seminal Vesiculitis: Inflammation of the seminal vesicles.

Sepsis: The presence of infectious organisms or their toxins in the blood or tissues that may be associated with fever, organ malfunction, abnormally low blood pressure, and even death.

Spermicide: Medications that kill sperm on contact. Usually used in conjunction with a diaphragm for birth control.

Stoma: For the purposes of this book, a surgically created opening on the skin where urine can exit the body.

Substance P: A small molecule found in certain nerve fibers. Substance P appears to stimulate inflammation and also functions in the transmission of pain within the nervous system.

Suprapubic: Above the pubic bone.

Supratrigonal Cystectomy: This is a form of partial bladder removal where almost the entire bladder is excised, leaving the very lower portion (the trigone) in place. A large piece of intestine usually is used to replace that portion of the bladder that has been excised (see figure 11A in chapter 8).

TENS (Transcutaneous Electrical Nerve Stimulation): A method of pain management using a low level of electrical stimulation applied to the body surface.

Trigone: The base of the bladder. *Trigonitis* is a nonspecific term denoting redness (possibly inflammation) in this region.

Uncomplicated Urinary Tract Infection: A urinary tract infection that is usually superficial, easily treated, and not associated with structural or functional abnormalities of the urinary tract.

Ureter: The two ureters transport urine from the kidneys down to the bladder. The small openings in the bladder where the urine enters are called the *ureteral orifices*.

Urethra: The tube that allows urine to exit the bladder. The opening where the urine comes out is called the *urethral meatus*.

Urethral Dilation: A "stretching" of the urethra performed by inserting an instrument called a urethral dilator. In many instances, progressively larger urethral dilators are inserted into the urethra until the desired degree of dilation is achieved.

Urethral Diverticulum: A small pouch or sac that connects to the urethra. Urine can fill this pouch, causing an uncomfortable sensation. More importantly, urine within the diverticulum can become infected and cause pain. (See figure 4 in chapter 2.)

Urethral Meatus: The opening of the urethra; located at the end of the penis in males and in the vagina in females.

Urethral Syndrome: A poorly understood condition marked by urinary urgency and frequency and urethral pain. Most patients also complain of urethral burning or burning while urinating. Urethral syndrome is believed by many to be a form of interstitial cystitis.

Urethral Stenosis: A narrowing of the urethra.

Urethritis: Inflammation of the urethra.

Urinalysis: A basic characterization of the urine including such parameters as pH, urine concentration, the presence or absence of blood, white blood cells, and sugar. Many urinalyses also include a microscopic review (called a *microscopic urinalysis*).

Urinary Diversion: A procedure in which the urine is diverted away from the bladder (the bladder can be left in place or removed).

Urinary Retention: The inability to empty the bladder. *Acute urinary retention* usually refers to the sudden inability to pass urine leading to symptoms of severe lower abdominal discomfort.

Urinary Sphincter: Two major sphincters controlling urination exist:

> 1. *Internal urinary sphincter*: This is muscle located at the neck of the bladder (the region where the urine exits). The sphincter is composed of muscle that is not under voluntary control.
>
> 2. *External urinary sphincter*: A complex group of muscles that allow the individual to start and stop the urinary stream. The external urinary sphincter is composed of muscle that normally can be relaxed or tightened at will.
>
> Both of these sphincters are responsible for the maintenance of urinary continence.

Urine Cytology: A urine test used to detect the presence of bladder cancers.

Urodynamics: Specialized testing of bladder function.

Uroflow: A test that demonstrates the characteristics of the urine flow.

Urothelium: The thin surface of the bladder that comes in contact with urine.

Vaginismus: Painful spasm of the vagina causing severe pain with sexual intercourse. Vaginismus appears to be caused by spasm of the pelvic floor muscles.

Vesical: Another term for the bladder.

Void: To urinate.

Voiding Diary: A self-assessment done to demonstrate patterns of urination.

Vulva: The external female genital region (see figure 3 in chapter 2) including the mons pubis, labia majora and minora, the vaginal vestibule, and the clitoris. The vestibule contains the urethral meatus, the opening of the vagina (the introitus), and numerous glands.

Vulvectomy: Excision of the vulva followed by surgical reconstruction of that region.

Vulvodynia: A general term literally meaning "vulvar pain." Vulvar pain can develop from many medical conditions such as estrogen loss and dermatological problems. In some instances, there is no apparent cause.

Resources

Urologic Organizations

Interstitial Cystitis Association
51 Monroe St., Suite 1402
Rockville, MD 20850
Toll free: 1-800-HELP-ICA: Tel: (301) 610-5300
Fax: (301) 610-5308
E-mail: Icinfo@ichelp.org   Web site: www.IChelp.org

American Foundation for Urologic Disease/The Bladder Health Council
1128 N. Charles Street
Baltimore, MD 21201
Toll-free: (800) 242-2383: Tel: (410) 468-1800
E-mail: admin@afud.org   Web site: www.afud.org

American Urological Association
1120 N. Charles Street
Baltimore, MD 21201
Tel: (410) 727-1100
Fax: (410) 468-1836
E-mail: aua@auanet.org   Web site: www.auanet.org

Interstitial Cystitis Network
4773 Sonoma Highway, PMB #125
Santa Rosa, CA 95409
Tel: (707) 538-9442
Fax: (707) 538-9444
E-mail: jill@ic-network.com   Web site: www.ic-network.org

National Association for Continence
P.O. Box 8306
Spartanburg, SC 29305-8306
Tel: (864) 579-7900
Fax: (864) 579-7902

National Bladder Foundation
P.O. Box 1095
Ridgefield, CT 06877
Tel: (203) 431-0005
Fax: (203) 431-0008
E-mail: debsla@aol.com   Web site: www.bladder.org

National Institute of Diabetes and Digestive and Kidney Diseases (NIDDK)
Office of Communications and Public Liaison, NIDDK, NIH
31 Center Drive, MSC 2560
Bethesda, MD 20892-2560
Web site: www.niddk.nih.gov

Prostatitis Foundation
1063 30th Street, Box 8
Smithshire, IL 61478
Toll-free: (888) 891-4200: Tel: (309) 325-7184
Web site: www.prostatitis.org

The Simon Foundation for Continence
P.O. Box 835-F
Wilmette, IL 60091
Toll-free: (800) 23-SIMON: Tel: (847) 864-3913
Fax: (847) 864-9758
Web site: www.simonfoundation.org

Society of Urologic Nurses and Associates
Web site: www.suna.org   E-mail: suna@ajj.org

www.clinicaltrials.gov
The National Institutes of Health, through its National Library of Medicine, has developed this web site called clinicaltrials.gov to provide patients, family members, and members of the public current information about clinical research studies, including IC.

International IC Organizations
Canada
Canadian Interstitial Cystitis Society (CICS)
Société Canadienne de la cystite interstitielle
Attn: Sandy McNicol, President

P.O. Box 28625
406 S. Willingdon Avenue
Burnaby, BC V5C 6J4 Canada
Phone: 250.758.3207
Fax: 250.758.4894
E-mail: smcnicol@pacificcoast.net

Germany

ICA Deutschland e.V.
Attn: Barbara Muendner-Hensen, Chair
Untere Burg 21
D-53881 Euskirchen Germany
Phone: +49.2251.76729
Fax: +49.2251.76729
Web site: http://www.ica-ev.de

Italy

Associazione Italiana Cistite Interstiziale
Attn: Loredana Nasta
Viale Glorioso 1
000153 Roma Italy
E-mail: AICI@mclink.it

The Netherlands

Interstitial Cystitis Patient's Association of the Netherlands (ICPA-NL)
Attn: Jane Meijlink, Chair
B.L.F. de Montignylan 73
3055 NA Rotterdam The Netherlands
Phone: +31.10.4613330
Fax: +31.10.2857158
E-mail: jane.meijlink@gironet.nl

New Zealand

New Zealand IC Support Group
Attn: Dot Milne, R.N.
Urology Support Services
P.O. Box 33-264
Christchurch New Zealand
Phone: +64.3.3294005

United Kingdom

Interstitial Cystitis Support Group (ICSG)
Attn: Anthony Walker, National Coordinator
76 High Street
Stony Stratford
Buckinghamshire MK11 1AH United Kingdom
Phone: +44.1908.569169
Fax: +44.1908.569169
E-mail: info@interstitialcystitis.co.uk
Web site: www.interstitialcystitis.co.uk

Organizations for IC-Related Conditions

Allergy and Asthma Network/Mothers of Asthmatics, Inc.
2751 Prosperity Ave., Suite 150
Fairfax, VA 22030-2709
Toll-free: (800) 878-4403: Tel: (703) 641-9595
Fax: (703) 575-7794   Web site: www.aanma.org

American Autoimmune Related Diseases Association, Inc.
22100 Gratiot Avenue
East Detroit, MI 48021
Toll-free: (810) 776-3900
Web site: www.aarda.org

American Council for Headache Education (ACHE)
19 Mantua Road
Mt. Royal, NJ 08061
Toll-free: (800) 255-2243: Tel: (609) 423-0258
Fax: (609) 423-0082
Web site: www.achenet.org

American Fibromyalgia Syndrome Association, Inc.
6389 E. Tanque Verde Rd., Suite D
Tucson, AZ 85715
Tel: (520) 773-1570
Fax: (520) 290-5550
Web site: www.afsafund.org

Arthritis Foundation
1330 West Peachtree
Atlanta, GA 30309
Toll-free: (800) 283-7800: Tel: (404) 872-7800
Web site: www.arthritis.org

Asthma & Allergy Foundation of America
1125 15th Street, NW Suite 502
Washington, DC 20005
Toll-free: (800) 727-8462: Tel: (202) 466-7643
Fax: (202) 466-8940
Web site: www.aafa.org

The CFIDS Association of America, Inc. (Chronic Fatigue & Immune Dysfunction Syndrome)
P. O. Box 220398
Charlotte, NC 28222-0398
Toll-free: (800) 44-CFIDS
Fax: (704) 365-9755
Resources: (704) 365-2343
E-mail: internet-info@cfids.org   Web site: www.cfids.org

Crohn's and Colitis Foundation of America, Inc.
National Headquarters
444 Park Ave. South, 11th Floor
New York, NY 10016
Toll-free: (800) 932-2423: Tel: (212) 779-4098
Web site: www.ccfa.org

Endometriosis Association, Inc.
8585 North 76th Place
Milwaukee, WI 53223
Toll-free: (800) 992-3636: Tel: (414) 355-2200
Fax: (414) 355-6065
Web site: www.endometriosisassn.org

Fibromyalgia Alliance of America
P.O. Box 21990
Columbus, OH 43221-0990
Tel: (614) 457-4222
Fax: (614) 457-2729
E-mail: FMSinfo@aol.com

Fibromyalgia Association of Greater Washington
13203 Valley Drive
Woodbridge, VA 22191-1531
Tel: (703) 551-4160
Fax: (703) 494-4103
E-mail: mail@fmagw.org   Web site: www.fmagw.org

The Fibromyalgia Network
P.O. Box 31750
Tucson, AZ 85751-1750
Toll-free: (800) 853-2929: Tel: (520) 290-6508

Fax: (520) 290-5550
Web site: www.fmnetnews.com

Fibromyalgia Wellness Newsletter (Arthritis Foundation)
P.O. Box 921907
Norcross, GA 30010-1907
Toll-free: (877) 775-0343

International Fibromyalgia Exchange
Deutsche Fibromyalgie-Vereinigung Postfach 1308
71536 Murrhardt, Germany
Internet: www.Weiss.de/Fibro.htm

International Foundation for Functional Gastrointestinal Disorders (IFFGD)
P.O. Box 17864
Milwaukee, WI 53217
Toll-free: (888) 964-2001: Tel: (414) 964-1799
E-mail: iffgd@iffgd.org   Web site: www.iffgd.org

Lupus Foundation of America
4 Research Place, Suite 180
Rockville, MD 20850-3226
Toll-free: (800) 558-0121: Tel: (301) 670-9292
Web site: www.lupus.org

Massachusetts CFIDS Association
P.O. Box 690305
Quincy, MA 02269-0305
Tel: (617) 471-5559
E-mail: webmaster@masscfids.org   Web site: www.masscfids.org

The Mastocytosis Society, Inc.
4771 Waynes Trace Road
Hamilton, OH 45011
Tel: (513) 726-4642
E-mail: LDB002@aol.com
Website: www.mastocytosis.org/www.mastocytosis.com

The National Headache Foundation
Toll-free: (888) NHF-5552
Fax: (773) 525-7357
Web site: www.headaches.org

National Sjogren's Syndrome Association
5815 North Black Canyon Highway, Suite 103
Phoenix, AZ 85015-2200
Toll-free: (800) 395-NSSA
Tel: (602) 516-0787
Fax: (602) 516-0111

National Vulvodynia Association
P.O. Box 4491
Silver Spring, MD 20914-4491
Tel: (301) 299-0775
Web site: www.nva.org

Sjogren's Syndrome Foundation
333 North Broadway
Jericho, NY 11753
Tel: (516) 933-6365
Web site: www.sjogrens.com

Vulvar Pain Foundation
203½ N. Main Street, Suite 203
Graham, NC
Tel: (336) 226-0704 (Tues. & Thurs.)
Fax: (336) 226-8518
Web site: www.vulvarpainfoundation.org

Pain Organizations

American Academy of Pain Management
13947 Mono Way #A
Sonora, CA 95370
Tel: (209) 533-9744
Web site: www.aapainmanage.org

American Academy of Pain Medicine
4700 W. Lake Avenue
Glenview, IL 60025
Toll-free: (847) 375-4731
Fax: (847) 375-6331
Web site: www.painmed.org

American Chronic Pain Association
P.O. Box 850
Rocklin, CA 95677
Tel: (916) 632-0922
Fax: (916) 632-3208
Web site: www.theacpa.org

American Pain Foundation
111 South Calvert Street, Suite 2700
Baltimore, MD 21202
E-mail: ampainfoun@aol.com   Web site: www.painfoundation.org

American Pain Society /International Association for the Study of Pain
4700 W. Lake Avenue
Glenview, IL 60025
Toll-free: (847) 375-4715
Fax: (847) 375-4777
E-mail: info@ampainsoc.org   Web site: www.ampainsoc.org

National Chronic Pain Outreach Association
P.O. Box 274
Millboro, VA 24460
Tel: (540) 997-5004
Fax: (540) 997-1305
Web site: http://www.paincare.org

National Foundation for the Treatment of Pain
1330 Skyline Drive #21
Monterey, CA 93940
Toll-free: (831) 655-8812
Fax: (831) 655-2823
Web site: www.paincare.org

Other Helpful Organizations

Reflex Sympathetic Dystrophy Syndrome Association of America
116 Haddon Avenue, Suite D
Haddonfield, NJ 08033
Tel: (609) 795-8845

TMJ Association (Temporal-Mandibular Joint Diseases)
P.O. Box 26770
Milwaukee, WI 54226
Tel: (414) 259-3223
Fax: (414) 259-8112
E-mail: info@tmj.org   Web site: www.tmj.org

United Ostomy Association
19772 McAuthur Blvd., Suite 120
Irvine, CA 92612
Toll-free: (800) 826-0826: Tel: (949) 660-8624
Fax: (949) 660-9262
Web site: www.uoa.org

Well Spouse Foundation
30 E. 40th Street PH
New York, NY 10018
Toll-free: (800) 838-0879: Tel: (212) 685-8815
Fax: (212) 685-8676
E-mail: wellspouse@aol.com

Special Concerns of Women

Centers for Disease Control & Prevention
Toll-free: (800) 311-3435
Web site: www.cdc.gov

Center for Patient Advocacy
Toll-free: (800) 846-7444
Web site: www.patientadvocacy.org

Food and Drug Administration
Toll-free: (888) 463-6332
Web site: www.fda.gov

HERS Foundation—Hysterectomy Educational Resources and Services
422 Bryn Mawr Avenue
Bala Cynwyd, PA 19004
Tel: (610) 667-7757
Fax: (610) 667-8096
Web site: www.nafc.org

National Center for Complementary and Alternative Medicine
Toll-free: (888) 644-6226
Web site: altmed.od.nih.gov/nccam

National Library of Medicine
Toll-free: (888) 346-3656
Web site: www.nlm.nih.gov

Society for the Advancement of Women's Health Research
1828 L Street, NW, Suite 625
Washington, DC 20036
Tel: (202) 223-8224
Fax: (202) 833-3472
E-mail: information@womens-health.org
Web site: www.womens-health.org

Disability/Social Security Information

Americans with Disabilities Act Information
Toll-free: (800) 514-0301 (Mon., Tues., Wed., Fri. 10:00 A.M. - 6:00 P.M., Thurs. 1:00 P.M. - 6:00 P.M.)

National Organization of Social Security Claimants' Representatives
6 Prospect Street
Midland Park, NJ 07432
Toll-free: (800) 431-2804: Tel: (201) 444-1415

Social Security Administration
Write or call your local office (look in your telephone book under
U.S. Government, Department of Health and Human Services) or call
1 (800) 234-5772 or visit their Web site at www.ssa.gov.

Cross-Cultural Health Organizations

The Center for Cross-Cultural Health
Suite W227, 410 Church Street, SE
Minneapolis, MN 55455
Tel: (612) 624-6930
Fax: (612) 625-1434
Web site: www.umn.edu/cch

National Asian Women's Health Organization
250 Montgomery Street, Suite 410
San Francisco, CA 94104
Tel: (415) 989-9747
Fax: (415) 989-9758

National Black Women's Health Project, Inc.
1211 Connecticut Avenue NW
Suite 310
Washington DC 20036
Tel: (202) 835-0117
Fax: (202) 833-8790
E-mail: nbwhpdc@aol.com

**National Coalition of Hispanic Health and Human Services
Organizations (COSSMHO)**
1501 16th Street NW
Washington DC 20036
Tel: (202) 387-5000

National Urban League
120 Wall Street
New York, NY 10005
Tel: (212) 558-5300
E-mail: info@nul.org
Web site: www.nul.org

References[*]

Introduction

Adams, R. D., V. Maurice, and A. H. Ropper. 1997a. Multiple Sclerosis and Allied Demyelinative Diseases. In *Principles of Neurology*, sixth edition. New York: McGraw-Hill, 902–927.

Adams, R. D., V. Maurice, and A. H. Ropper. 1997b. The Muscular Dystrophies. In *Principles of Neurology*, sixth edition. New York: McGraw-Hill, 1414–1431.

Curhan, G. C., F. E. Speizer, D. J. Hunter, S. G. Curhan, and M. J. Stampfer. 1999. Epidemiology of Interstitial Cystitis: A Population-based Study. *Journal of Urology* 161:549–552.

Gladman, D. D., and M. C. Hochberg. 1999. The Epidemiology of Systemic Lupus, Erythematosus. In *Systemic Lupus Erythematosus*, third edition, edited by R. G. Lahita. San Diego, CA: Academic Press, 537–540.

Rodgers, G. M., and C. S. Greenberg. 1999. Inherited Coagulation Disorders. In *Wintrobe's Clinical Hematology*, tenth edition, edited by G. R. Lee, J. Foerster, J. Lukens, F. Paresky, J. P. Greer, and G. M. Rodgers. Baltimore: William and Wilkens, 1682–1687.

Chapter 1

Hunner, G. L. 1915. A Rare Type of Bladder Ulcer in Women: Report of Cases. *Transactions of the Southern Surgery and Gynecological Association* 27:247–292.

Koziol, J. A., D. C. Clark, R. F. Gittes, and E. M. Tan. 1993. The Natural History of Interstitial Cystitis: A Survey of 374 Patients. *Journal of Urology. 149:465–469.*

---

[*] For additional bibliographic information, please write to the author care of New Harbinger Publications.

Skene, A. J. C. 1887. *Diseases of Bladder and Urethra in Women*. New York: Wm. Wood, 167.

Chapter 2

Erickson, D. R., S. Mast, S. Ordille, and V. P. Bhavanandan. 1996. Urinary Epitectin (MUC-1 Glycoprotein) in the Menstrual Cycle and Interstitial Cystitis. *Journal of Urology* 156:938–942.

Erickson, D. R., M. Sheykhnazari, S. Ordille, and V. P. Bhavanandan. 1998. Increased Urinary Hyaluronic Acid and Interstitial Cystitis. *Journal of Urology* 160:1282–1284.

Hanno, P. M., J. R. Landis, Y. Matthews-Cook, J. Kusek, L. Nyber, Jr., and the Interstitial Cystitis Database Study Group. 1999. The Diagnosis of Interstitial Cystitis Revisited: Lessons Learned from the National Institutes of Health Interstitial Cystitis Database Study. *Journal of Urology* 161:553–557.

Hurst, R. E., C. L. Parsons, J. B. Roy, and J. L.Young.1993. Urinary Glycosaminoglycan Excretion as a Laboratory Marker in the Diagnosis of Interstitial Cystitis. *Journal of Urology* 149:31–35.

Keay, S., C. O. Zhang, M. K. Hise, J. R. Hebel, S. C. Jacobs, C. Gordon, K. Whitmore, S. Bodison, N. Gordon, and J. W. Warren. 1998. A Diagnostic In Vitro Urine Assay for Interstitial Cystitis. *Urology* 52(6):974–8.

Moskowitz, M. O., D. Shupp-Byrne, H. J. Callahan, C. L. Parsons, E. Valderrama, and R. M. Moldwin. 1994. Decreased Expression of a Glycoprotein Component of Bladder Surface Mucin (GP1) in Interstitial Cystitis. *Journal of Urology* 151:343–345.

Teichman, J. M. H., and B. J. Neilsen-Omeis. 1999. Potassium Leak Test Predicts Outcome in Interstitial Cystitis. *Journal of Urology* 161:1791–1796.

Chapter 3

Anderson, J. B., F. Parivar, G. Lee, T. B. Wallington, A. G. MacIver, R. A. Bradbrook, and J. C Gingell. 1989. The Enigma of Interstitial Cystitis—An Autoimmune Disease? *British Journal of Urology* 63:58–63.

Chen Y., R. Varghese, J. Lehrer, S. Tillem, R. Moldwin, and L. Kushner. 1999. Urinary Substance P Is Elevated in Women with Interstitial Cystitis. *Journal of Urology* 161:26.

Dixon, J. S., M. Holm-Bentzen, C. J. Gilpin, J. A. Gosling, E. Bostofte, T. Hald, and S. Larsen. 1986. Electron Microscopic Investigation of the Bladder Urothelium and Glycocalyx in Patients with Interstitial Cystitis. *Journal of Urology* 135:621–625.

Elgavish, A., A. Pattanaik, K. Lloyd, and R. Reed. 1997. Evidence for Altered Proliferative Ability of Progenitors of Urothelial Cells in Interstitial Cystitis. *Journal of Urology. 158:248–252.*

———. 1994. Integrin-mediated Adhesive Properties of Uroepithelial Cells Are Inhibited by Treatment with Bacterial Toxins. *America Journal of Physiology* 266:C1552–C1559.

Holm-Bentzen M., J. Nordling, and T. Hald. 1990. Etiologic and Pathogenetic Theories in Interstitial Cystitis. In: *Interstitial Cystitis*, edited by P. M

Hanno, D. R. Staskin, R. J Krane, and A. J. Wein. London: Springer-Verlag, 63–77.

Irwin, P., and N. T. M. Galloway. 1993. Impaired Bladder Perfusion in Interstitial Cystitis. *Journal of Urology* 149:890–892.

Kastrup, J., J. Hald, L. Larsen, and V. G. Nielsen. 1983. Histamine Content and Mast Cell Count in Patients with Interstitial Cystitis and Other Types of Chronic Cystitis. *British Journal of Urology* 55:495–500.

Lilly, J. D., and C. L. Parsons. 1990. Bladder Surface Glycosaminoglycans Is a Human Epithelial Permeability Barrier. *Surgery, Gynecology and Obstetrics* 171:493–496.

Moskowitz, M. O., D. Shupp-Byrne, H. J. Callahan, C. L. Parsons, E. Valderrama, and R. M. Moldwin. 1994. Decreased Expression of a Glycoprotein Component of Bladder Surface Mucin (GP1) in Interstitial Cystitis. *Journal of Urology* 151:343–345.

Pang, X., J. Marchand, G. R. Sant, R. M. Kream, and T. C. Theoharides. 1993. Increased Numbers of Substance P (SP): Positive Nerve Fibers Associated with Bladder Mast Cells in Interstitial Cystitis (IC). Research Symposium on Interstitial Cystitis, A Century of Awareness, A Decade of Progress, Orlando, FL. Oct. 8-9, p. 44.

Pontari, M. A., P. M. Hanno, and M. R. Ruggieri. 1999. Comparison of Bladder Blood Flow in Patients With and Without Interstitial Cystitis. *Journal of Urology* 162(2):330–334.

Silk, M. R. 1970. Bladder Antibodies in Interstitial Cystitis. *Journal of Urology* 103:307-309.

Chapter 4

Alagiri, M., S. Chottiner, V. Ratner, D. Slade, and P. Hanno. 1997. Interstitial Cystitis: Unexplained Associations with Other Chronic Disease and Pain Syndromes. *Urology* (Suppl. 5A)49:52–57.

Avorn, J., M. Monane, J. H. Gurwitz, R. J. Glynn, I. Choodnovskiy, and L. A. Lipsitz. 1994. Reduction of Bacteriuria and Pyuria After Ingestion of Cranberry Juice. *Journal of the American Medical Association* 271:751–754.

Baggish, M. S., E. H. M. Sze, and R. Johnson. 1997. Urinary Oxalate Excretion and Its Role in Vulvar Pain Syndrome. *American Journal of Obstetrics and Gynecology* 177:509–511.

Barnett, B. J., and D. S. Stephens. 1997. Urinary Tract Infection: An Overview. *American Journal of Medical Science* 314:245–249.

Bohm-Starke, N., M. Hilliges, C. Falconer, and E. Rylander. 1998. Increased Intraepithelial Innervation in Women with Vulvar Vestibulitis Syndrome. *Gynecol. Obstet. Invest.* 46:256–260.

Boreham, P. 1984. Cryosurgery for the Urethral Syndrome. *Journal of the Royal Society of Medicine* 77:111–113.

Deluze C., L. Bosia, A. Zirbs, A. Chantraine, and T. L. Vischer. 1992. Electroacupuncture in Fibromyalgia: Results of a Controlled Trial. *British Medical Journal* 305:1249–1252.

Foxman, B., and R. R. Frerichs. 1985. Epidemiology of Urinary Tract Infection: Diaphragm Use and Sexual Intercourse. *American Journal of Public Health* 75:1308–1313.

Gittes, R. F., and R. Nakamura. 1996. Female Urethral Syndrome. *Western Journal of Medicine* 164:435–438.

Glazer, H. I., G. Rodke, C. Swencionis, R. Hertz, and A. W. Young. 1995. Treatment of Vulvar Vestibulitis Syndrome with Electromyographic Feedback of Pelvic Floor Musculature. *Journal of Reproductive Medicine* 40:283–290.

Glazer, H. I. 1998. Electromyographic Comparisons of the Pelvic Floor in Women with Dysesthetic Vulvodynia and Asymptomatic Women. *Journal of Reproductive Medicine* 43:959–962.

Golding, J. M., S. C. Wilsnack, and L. A. Learman. 1998. Prevalence of Sexual Assault History Among Women in Common Gynecological Symptoms. *American Journal of Obstetrics and Gynecology* 179:1013–1019.

Hand, J. R. 1949. Interstitial Cystitis: Report of 223 Cases. *Journal of Urology* 61:291–310.

Lemack, G. E., B. Foster, and P. E. Zimmern. 1999. Urethral Dilation in Women: A Questionnaire-based Analysis of Practice Patterns. *Urology* 54:37–43.

Ridley, C. M. 1998. Vulvodynia: Theory and Management. *Derm. Clinics* 16:775–778.

Rutherford, A. J., K. Hinshaw, D. M. Essenhigh, and D. E. Neal. 1988. Urethral Dilatation Compared with Cystoscopy Alone in the Treatment of Women with Recurrent Frequency and Dysuria. *British Journal of Urology* 61:500–504.

Sand, P. K., L. W. Bowen, D. R. Ostergard, A. Bent, and R. Panganiban. 1989. Cryosurgery Versus Dilatation and Massage for the Management of Recurrent Urethral Syndrome. *Journal of Reproductive Medicine* 34:499–504.

Schmidt, D. R., and A. E. Sobota. 1988. An Examination of the Anti-Adherence Activity of Cranberry Juice on Urinary and Nonurinary Bacterial Isolates. *Microbios* UK. 55:173–181.

Solomons, C., M. H. Melmed, and S. M. Heitler. 1991. Calcium Citrate for Vulvar Vestibulitis: A Case Report. *Journal of Reproductive Medicine* 36:879–882.

Chapter 5

Badenoch, A. 1971. Chronic Interstitial Cystitis. *British Journal of Urology* 43:718.

Ehren, I., A. Hosseini, J. O. N. Lundberg, and N. P. Wiklund. 1999. Nitric Oxide: A Useful Gas in the Detection of Lower Urinary Tract Inflammation. *Journal of Urology* 162:327–329.

Hanno, P. M., and A. J. Wein. 1991. Conservative Therapy of Interstitial Cystitis. *Seminars in Urology* 9(2):143–147.

Fleischmann, J. D., H. N. Huntley, W. B. Singleton, and D. B. Wentworth. 1991. Clinical and Immunological Response to Nifedipine for the Treatment of Interstitial Cystitis. *Journal of Urology* 146:1235–1239.

Korting, G. E., S. D. Smith, M. A. Wheeler, and R. M. Weiss. 1999. A Randomized Double-Blind Trial of Oral L-arginine in the Treatment of Interstitial Cystitis. *Journal of Urology* 161(2):558–565.

Seshadri, P. 1994. Cimetidine in the Treatment of Interstitial Cystitis. *Urology* 44(4):614–616.

Smith, S. D., M. A. Wheeler, H. E. Foster, Jr., and R. M. Weiss. 1997. Improvement in Interstitial Cystitis Symptom Scores During Treatment with Oral L-arginine. *Journal of Urology* 158:703–708.

Chapter 6

Cruz, F., M. Guimarães, C. Silva, M. Edite Rio, A. Coimbra, and M. Reis. 1997. Desensitization of Bladder Sensory Fibers by Intravesical Capsaicin Has Long-Lasting Clinical and Urodynamic Effects in Patients with Hyperactive and Hypersensitive Bladder Dysfunction. *Journal of Urology* 157:585–589.

Edwards, L., J. E. Bucknall, and C. Makin. 1986. Interstitial Cystitis: Possible Cause and Clinical Study of Sodium Cromoglycate. *British Journal of Urology* 58:95–96.

Flood, H. D., D. A. Shupp-Byrne, P. Rivas, J. McCue, J. A. Sedor, M. B. Crewalk, et. al. 1997. Intravesical Capsaicin for Interstitial Cystitis *Journal of Urology* 157:254.

Fowler, J. E. 1981. Prospective Study of Dimethyl Sulfoxide in the Treatment of Suspected Early Interstitial Cystitis. *Urology* 18:21–26.

Ghoniem, G. M., D. McBride, O. P. Sood, and V. Lewis. 1993. Clinical Experience with Multiagent Intravesical Therapy in Interstitial Cystitis Patients Unresponsive to Single-Agent Therapy. *World Journal of Urology* 11:178–182.

Jespersen, J., and T. Astrup. 1985. Chronic Interstitial Cystitis and Subcutaneous Heparin. *Lancet* (Nov. 2) 2:1010–1011.

Kennelly, M. J., and J. W. Konnak. 1995. Intravesical Cromolyn Sodium for the Treatment of Interstitial Cystitis—A Double-Blind Placebo Controlled Pilot Study. Research Symposium on Interstitial Cystitis, Jan. 9-11, National Institutes of Health, Bethesda, MD, p. 64.

La Rock, D. R., and G. Sant. 1997. Intravesical Therapies for Interstitial Cystitis. In *Interstitial Cystitis,* edited by G. R. Sant. Philadelphia: Lippincott-Raven Publishers, 247–255.

Lazzeri, M., P. Beneforte, D. Turini, M. Spinelli, and A. Zaneilo. 1998. Intravesical Resiaferitoxin for the Treatment of Detrusor Hyperreflexia Refractory to Capcaisin. *Journal of Urology* 159:83 (Abstract 316).

Lose, G., J. Jesperson, B. Frandsen, J. C. Hojensgard, and T. Astrup. 1985. Subcutaneous Heparin in the Treatment of Interstitial Cystitis. *Scandinavian Journal of Urology and Nephrology* 19: 27–29.

Maggi, C. A., G. Barbanti, P. Santicioli, P. Beneforte, D. Misuri, A. Meli, and D. Turini. 1989. Cystometric Evidence That Capsaicin-Sensitive Nerves Modulate the Afferent Branch of Micturition Reflex in Humans. *Journal of Urology* 149:150–154.

Messing, E. M., and T. A. Stamey. 1978. Interstitial Cystitis: Early Diagnosis, Pathology, and Treatment. *Urology* 12:381–392.

Morales, A., L. Emerson, and J. C. Nickel. 1997. Intravesical Hyaluronic Acid in the Treatment of Refractory Interstitial Cystitis. *Urology* 49 (5A Supp.):111–113.

Parsons, C. L., T. Housley, J. D. Schmidt, and D. Lebow. 1993. Treatment of Interstitial Cystitis with Intravesical Heparin. Research Symposium on Interstitial Cystitis, A Century of Awareness, A Decade of Progress, Orlando, Fl. Oct. 8-9, p. 48.

Perez-Marrero, R., L. E. Emerson, and J. T. Feltis. 1988. A Controlled Study of Dimethyl Sulfoxide in Interstitial Cystitis. *Journal of Urology* 140:36–39.

Peters, K., A. C. Diokno, B. W. Steinert, and J. A. Gonzalez. 1998. The Efficacy of Bacillus Calmette-Guerin in the Treatment of Interstitial Cystitis: Long-Term Follow-up. *Journal of Urology* 159: 1483–1487.

Porru, D., G. Campus, D. Tudino, E. Valdes, A. Vespa, R. M. Scarpa, and E. Usai. 1997. Results of Treatment of Refractory Interstitial Cystitis with Intravesical Hyaluronic Acid. *Urology International* 59:26–29.

Riedl, C. R., M. Knoll, E. Plas, and H. Pflüger. 1998. Intravesical Electromotive Drug Administration Technique: Preliminary Results and Side Effects. *Journal of Urology* 159:1851–1856.

Stewart, B. H., L. Persky, and W. S. Kiser. 1968. The Use of Dimethyl Sulfoxide (DMSO) in the Treatment of Interstitial Cystitis. *Journal of Urology* 98:671–672.

Wishard, W. N., M. H. Nourse, and J. H. O. Mertz. 1957. The Use of Clorpactin WCS 90 Therapy for Interstitial Cystitis. *Journal of Urology* 77:420–423.

Chapter 7

Hanash, K. A., and T. L. Pool. 1969. Interstitial Cystitis in Men. *Journal of Urology* 102:427–428.

Messing, E. M. 1987. The Diagnosis of Interstitial Cystitis. *Urology* 29 (Suppl. 4):4–7.

Miller, J. L., I. Rothman, T. G. Bavendam, and R. E. Berger. 1995. Prostatodynia and Interstitial Cystitis: One and the Same? *Urology* 45:587–590.

Nickel, J. C., J. Downey, J. Clark, H. Ceri, and M. Olson. 1995. Antibiotic Pharmacokinetics in the Inflamed Prostate. *Journal of Urology* 158:527–529.

Siroky, M. B., I. Goldstein, and R. J. Krane. 1981. Functional Voiding Disorders in Men. *Journal of Urology* 126:200–204.

Chapter 8

MacDermott, J. P., G. L. Charpied, H. Tesluk, and A. R. Stone. 1990. Recurrent Interstitial Cystitis Following Cystoplasty: Fact or Fiction? *Journal of Urology* 144:37–40.

Moldwin, R. M., and F. Mendelowitz. 1993. Pelvic Floor Dysfunction and Interstitial Cystitis. Research Symposium on Interstitial Cystitis, A Century of Awareness, A Decade of Progress, Orlando, FL. Oct. 8-9, p. 46.

Chapter 9

Goodwin, A. J., and M. E. Agronin. 1997. *A Woman's Guide to Overcoming Sexual Fear and Pain*. Oakland, CA: New Harbinger Publications.

Chapter 10

Fall, M., C. A. Carlsson, and B. E. Erlandson. 1980. Electrical Simulation in Interstitial Cystitis. *Journal of Urology* 123:192–195.

Geirsson, G., Y. H. Wang, S. Lindstrom, and M. Fall. 1993. Traditional Acupuncture and Electrical Stimulation of the Posterior Tibial Nerve: A Trial in Chronic Interstitial Cystitis. *Scandanavian Journal of Urology and Nephrology* 27:67–70.

Gillespie, L. 1986. *You Don't Have to Live with Cystitis!* New York: Avon Books, 244.

Glazer, H. I., G. Rodke, C. Swencionis, R. Hertz, and A. W. Young. 1995. Treatment of Vulvar Vestibulitis Syndrome with Electromyographic Feedback of Pelvic Floor Musculature. *Journal of Reproductive Medicine* 40:283–290.

Helms, J. M. 1987. Acupuncture for the Management of Primary Dysmenorrhea. *Obstetrics and Gynecology* 69:51–56.

Koziol, J. A., D. C. Clark, R. F. Gittes, and E. M. Tan. 1993. The Natural History of Interstitial Cystitis: A Survey of 374 Patients. *Journal of Urology 149:465–469.*

Laumann, Beverly. No date. *A Taste of the Good Life: A Cookbook for the Interstitial Cystitis Diet.* P. O. Box 402, Tustin, CA 92781: Freeman Family Trust Publications. Fall, M. 1987. Transcutaneous Electrical Nerve Stimulation in Interstitial Cystitis. *Urology* (Suppl.) 29:40–42.

Mendelowitz, F., and R. Moldwin. 1997. Complementary Approaches in the Management of Interstitial Cystitis. In *Interstitial Cystitis*, edited by G. R. Sant. Philadelphia: Lippincott-Raven Publishers, 235–239.

Shoskes, D. A., S. I. Zeitlin, A. Shahed, and J. Rajfer. 1999. Quercetin in Men with Category III Chronic Prostatitis: A Preliminary Prospective, Double-Blind, Placebo-Controlled Trial. *Urology* 54: 960–963.

Spanos, C., X. Pang, K. Ligris, R. Letourneau, L. Alferes, N. Alexacos, G. R. Sant, and T. C. Theoharides. 1997. Stress-Induced Bladder Mast Cell Activation: Implications for Interstitial Cystitis. *Journal of Urology* 157:669–72.

Chapter 11

Alagiri M., S. Chottiner, V. Ratner, D. Slade, and P. M. Hanno. 1997. Interstitial Cystitis: Unexplained Associations with Other Chronic Diseases and Pain Syndromes. *Urology* 49 (Supp. 5a) 52–57.

Campbell's Urology. 1979. Edited by J. H. Harrison, R. F. Gittes, A. D. Perlmutter, et al. Philadelphia: W. B. Saunders, 1906–1907.

Harrison, J. H., R. F. Gittes, A. D. Perlmutter, et al., eds. 1979. *Campbell's Urology*. Philadelphia: W. B. Saunders. 1906-1907.

Ratner, V., and D. Slade. 1997. A Woman's Health Perspective. In *Interstitial Cystitis*, edited by G. R. Sant. Philadelphia: Lippincott-Raven Publishers.

Wells, Susan Milstrey. 1998. *A Delicate Balance: Living Successfully with Chronic Illness*. New York: Insight Books.

Index

More New Harbinger Titles

BREAKING THE BONDS OF IRRITABLE BOWEL SYNDROME

Shows how to identify troublesome foods, develop strategies for managing flare-ups, and challenge the thoughts and emotional reactions that prevent you from recovering. *Item IBS $14.95*

HIGH ON STRESS

A Woman's Guide to Optimizing the Stress in Her Life

Helps you rethink the role of stress in your life, rework your responses to it, and find ways to boost the positive impact that it can have on your well-being. *Item HOS $13.95*

PERIMENOPAUSE

Changes in Women's Health After 35

Perimenopause begins with subtle physiological changes in the mid-thirties and forties, and it can encompass a bewildering array of symptoms. This self-care guide helps you cope and assure your health and vitality in the years ahead. *Item PERI $13.95*

THE ENDOMETRIOSIS SURVIVAL GUIDE

Clears up the myths, evaluates the latest treatment options, addresses concerns about infertility, and takes a balanced look at traditional and alternative coping strategies. *Item ENDO $13.95*

OVERCOMING REPETITIVE MOTION INJURIES THE ROSSITER WAY

This system of easy-to-learn stretches has brought pain relief to thousands who suffer from carpal tunnel syndrome and other repetitive motion injuries and everyday aches and pain. *Item ROSS $15.95*

THE FIBROMYALGIA ADVOCATE

Shows you how to assemble a functional health care team, deal with the legal aspects of the health care system, and fight for your right to receive effective care for fibromyalgia and the related condition of myofascial pain syndrome. *Item FMA $18.95*

Call **toll-free 1-800-748-6273** to order. Have your Visa or Mastercard number ready. Or send a check for the titles you want to New Harbinger Publications, 5674 Shattuck Avenue, Oakland, CA 94609. Include $3.80 for the first book and 75¢ for each additional book to cover shipping and handling. (California residents please include appropriate sales tax.) Allow four to six weeks for delivery.

Prices subject to change without notice.

Some Other New Harbinger Self-Help Titles

Multiple Chemical Sensitivity: A Survival Guide, $16.95
Dancing Naked, $14.95
Why Are We Still Fighting, $15.95
From Sabotage to Success, $14.95
Parkinson's Disease and the Art of Moving, $15.95
A Survivor's Guide to Breast Cancer, $13.95
Men, Women, and Prostate Cancer, $15.95
Make Every Session Count: Getting the Most Out of Your Brief Therapy, $10.95
Virtual Addiction, $12.95
After the Breakup, $13.95
Why Can't I Be the Parent I Want to Be?, $12.95
The Secret Message of Shame, $13.95
The OCD Workbook, $18.95
Tapping Your Inner Strength, $13.95
Binge No More, $14.95
When to Forgive, $12.95
Practical Dreaming, $12.95
Healthy Baby, Toxic World, $15.95
Making Hope Happen, $14.95
I'll Take Care of You, $12.95
Survivor Guilt, $14.95
Children Changed by Trauma, $13.95
Understanding Your Child's Sexual Behavior, $12.95
The Self-Esteem Companion, $10.95
The Gay and Lesbian Self-Esteem Book, $13.95
Making the Big Move, $13.95
How to Survive and Thrive in an Empty Nest, $13.95
Living Well with a Hidden Disability, $15.95
Overcoming Repetitive Motion Injuries the Rossiter Way, $15.95
What to Tell the Kids About Your Divorce, $13.95
The Divorce Book, Second Edition, $15.95
Claiming Your Creative Self: True Stories from the Everyday Lives of Women, $15.95
Six Keys to Creating the Life You Desire, $19.95
Taking Control of TMJ, $13.95
What You Need to Know About Alzheimer's, $15.95
Winning Against Relapse: A Workbook of Action Plans for Recurring Health and Emotional Problems, $14.95
Facing 30: Women Talk About Constructing a Real Life and Other Scary Rites of Passage, $12.95
The Worry Control Workbook, $15.95
Wanting What You Have: A Self-Discovery Workbook, $18.95
When Perfect Isn't Good Enough: Strategies for Coping with Perfectionism, $13.95
Earning Your Own Respect: A Handbook of Personal Responsibility, $12.95
High on Stress: A Woman's Guide to Optimizing the Stress in Her Life, $13.95
Infidelity: A Survival Guide, $13.95
Stop Walking on Eggshells, $14.95
Consumer's Guide to Psychiatric Drugs, $16.95
The Fibromyalgia Advocate: Getting the Support You Need to Cope with Fibromyalgia and Myofascial Pain, $18.95
Healing Fear: New Approaches to Overcoming Anxiety, $16.95
Working Anger: Preventing and Resolving Conflict on the Job, $12.95
Sex Smart: How Your Childhood Shaped Your Sexual Life and What to Do About It, $14.95
You Can Free Yourself From Alcohol & Drugs, $13.95
Amongst Ourselves: A Self-Help Guide to Living with Dissociative Identity Disorder, $14.95
Healthy Living with Diabetes, $13.95
Dr. Carl Robinson's Basic Baby Care, $10.95
Better Boundries: Owning and Treasuring Your Life, $13.95
Goodbye Good Girl, $12.95
Fibromyalgia & Chronic Myofascial Pain Syndrome, $19.95
The Depression Workbook: Living With Depression and Manic Depression, $17.95
Self-Esteem, Second Edition, $13.95
Angry All the Time: An Emergency Guide to Anger Control, $12.95
When Anger Hurts, $13.95
Perimenopause, $16.95
The Relaxation & Stress Reduction Workbook, Fourth Edition, $17.95
The Anxiety & Phobia Workbook, Second Edition, $18.95
I Can't Get Over It, A Handbook for Trauma Survivors, Second Edition, $16.95
Messages: The Communication Skills Workbook, Second Edition, $15.95
Thoughts & Feelings, Second Edition, $18.95
Depression: How It Happens, How It's Healed, $14.95
The Deadly Diet, Second Edition, $14.95
The Power of Two, $15.95

Call **toll free, 1-800-748-6273**, or log on to our online bookstore at **www.newharbinger.com** to order. Have your Visa or Mastercard number ready. Or send a check for the titles you want to New Harbinger Publications, Inc., 5674 Shattuck Ave., Oakland, CA 94609. Include $3.80 for the first book and 75¢ for each additional book, to cover shipping and handling. (California residents please include appropriate sales tax.) Allow two to five weeks for delivery.

Prices subject to change without notice.